Foods That COMBAT DIABETES

The Nutritional Way to Wellness

Maggie Greenwood-Robinson, Ph.D.

A Lynn Sonberg Book

HARPER

An Imprint of HarperCollinsPublishers

HARPER

An Imprint of HarperCollins*Publishers*
10 East 53rd Street
New York, New York 10022-5299

First Harper paperback printing: January 2008

HarperCollins® and Harper® are registered trademarks of Harper-Collins Publishers.

Printed in the United States of America

Visit Harper paperbacks on the World Wide Web at
www.harpercollins.com

10   9   8   7   6   5   4   3

ACKNOWLEDGMENTS

Special thanks to the following people for their work and contributions to this book: my agent, Madeleine Morel, 2M Communications, Ltd.; Lynn Sonberg of Lynn Sonberg Books; and the staff at Avon Books.

CONTENTS

CHAPTER 1

EAT TO DEFEAT DIABETES

In an ideal world, diabetes would not exist. In the real world, of course, diabetes is the nation's third leading cause of death, affecting 7 percent of our population. Recently, scientists have made huge strides in treating diabetes, from developing better drugs to launching an inhaled form of insulin, but one therapy stands head and shoulders above everything else: food.

The impact of food on diabetes was made crystal clear in a study of Pima Indians in Arizona and Mexico. As Native Americans, these people have a statistically higher risk of diabetes than most other ethnic groups. Yet researchers discovered that the Mexican Pima Indians, who live without so-called modern conveniences and eat a traditional, low-fat diet, have a much lower rate of the disease (6.5 percent) than the Arizona Pima Indians, who enjoy modern conveniences, eat fatty, processed foods, and have an alarming 38.2 percent diabetes rate.

Recently, I met a gentleman, Ben, who was being treated for type 2 diabetes. He was taking six different oral diabetes drugs and was about to be put on injectable insulin because, despite the drug therapy, he could not get his blood sugar under control. It soared at around 290 (which is extremely high). Ben decided to get serious about nutrition—I mean really serious—and use food to help his body heal. Within two weeks, his blood sugar stabilized at 100! That's normal and a reading doctors like to see. There was no need for Ben to take insulin, and he was able to reduce his oral medications to only one pill. Amazing? Yes. Miraculous? Not really. Food really is that powerful when it comes to controlling, and often, reversing, diabetes.

Diabetes, of course, is a disease of metabolism: Something goes haywire in the way the body processes food. When a healthy person eats carbohydrates (like bread, potatoes, or cereal), they get broken down into sugar and sent into the bloodstream. Insulin, a hormone produced by the pancreas, then acts as a delivery system, moving the sugar from your blood into your cells, where it is burned for fuel. When diabetes strikes, the pancreas either stops making insulin (type 1 diabetes), or the body cells become insulin-resistant and "reject delivery" of all or most of the sugar (type 2 diabetes). Either way, sugar builds up in the blood, the body doesn't get enough fuel, and complications such as heart disease, kidney disease, nerve damage, and eye disease can result.

Even so, you can get diabetes under control. Not only that, you can prevent it. Medical researchers and physicians have now recognized a diagnosable condition called *prediabetes*, which, if treated early with diet, exercise, and other lifestyle changes, can be stopped in its tracks. Prediabetes is a condition that raises the risk of developing type 2 diabetes, heart disease, and stroke. People with prediabetes have blood glucose levels higher than normal but not high enough to be classified as diabetes. Your physician can tell if you're prediabetic by running a number of routine tests, including blood sugar tests, usually at your annual physical. If he or she says you're prediabetic, making some fairly simple tweaks in the way you eat can turn this situation around dramatically. This book can help you do that.

Lots of accumulating research shows that you can reverse the course of prediabetes and prevent type 2 diabetes with diet and other lifestyle adjustments. Some of the most dramatic proof is found in the Diabetes Prevention Program (DPP). The DPP includes lifestyle guidelines intended to help people lose 7 percent of their initial body weight through restricting calories and exercising moderately for 150 minutes a week. Participants in the 16-week program learned to set specific goals for nutrition, exercise, and weight loss. Most of the 1,000 participants were successful and dropped their risk of diabetes by 58 percent. The drop in risk was even greater—71 percent—among people older than age 60. This all goes to show that type 2 diabetes is a lifestyle disease, but one that can be treated with lifestyle changes.

Insulin is the main therapy for type 1 diabetes, because people with this version of diabetes need insulin to survive. Though it plays a secondary role in type 1 diabetes, nutrition is nonetheless very important, since it can help control blood sugar highs that are at the root of all diabetic complications.

Thankfully, as serious as diabetes is, it does not have to be life-threatening. You can live with it, and you can live *well* with it. The keys to managing diabetes are a healthful diet, regular exercise, stress management, and medication if your doctor prescribes it. So given the tremendous impact nutrition has on preventing and treating diabetes, it is not surprising that there are specific foods that are particularly healing. This book is an overview of foods that truly do combat diabetes.

Diabetes-Fighting Carbs

Carbohydrates like breads, cereals, and potatoes are energy foods. During digestion, they are changed into glucose (blood sugar), which circulates in your blood and is used as fuel for the red blood cells and your central nervous system. Glucose not used right away is stored in the liver and muscles as glycogen, which provides an additional reservoir for energy.

Carbohydrates play an important role in preventing and controlling diabetes, as long as *you choose the right types of carbohydrates.* This is where food choice becomes all-important to your success. Carbohydrates are classified in various ways. One classification sorts them as either *simple* or *complex.* Simple sugars are found in candies, syrups, many fruits and fruit juices, and processed foods, and complex carbohydrates are found in whole grains, beans, fruits, and vegetables. This classification is based on the molecular structure of the carbohydrate, with simple carbohydrates constructed of either single or double molecules of sugar, and complex carbohydrates made of multiple numbers of sugar molecules. It's smart to cut back on your overall intake of simple sugars such as cookies, cake, and the like because they raise blood sugar, which can jeopardize your overall health if you have diabetes. Sugar is found in many unexpected places, like breads, pasta sauces, and salad dressings. To make matters worse, sugar goes by a number of different names, including fructose, maltose, sucrose, and glucose. A watchful eye when reading nutrition labels is your best defense against this foe.

So if you have diabetes, swap simple carbohydrates for complex carbohydrates. Complex carbohydrates are a healthier choice, because they are higher in healing nutrients such as fiber, vitamins, minerals, antioxidants, and phytochemicals. Antioxidants are nutrients that fight "free radicals," unstable molecules that damage otherwise healthy cells, and phytochemicals are naturally occurring substances in foods that fight disease.

Fiber: A Healing Carbohydrate

When you eat complex carbohydrates, you automatically get more of a vital substance called fiber. Fiber is the non-digestible carbohydrate in plant foods that keeps you regular, and has a long list of other impressive health benefits, particularly if you have diabetes or want to prevent it. Fiber helps keep your blood sugar under better control, without you having to constantly work at it or make yourself crazy. The reason is that high-fiber foods break down into glucose more gradually and are absorbed more slowly into the bloodstream. They stabilize your blood sugar and do not cause post-meal surges. Shoot for a goal of 25 to 35 grams of fiber daily. (For a list of fiber-rich foods, refer to the table below.) The information in this book will help you tally up your daily fiber quota.

In addition, if you have type 2 diabetes and take medicine, you may be able to eliminate or reduce your medication requirement by eating a diet high in natural carbohydrates and fiber. Case in point: In one study, 701 type 2 diabetics were asked to follow a high-fiber diet and exercise daily. Of these people, 207 were taking oral drugs to control their blood sugar levels, and 214 were using supplemental insulin. The rest were not on medication of any kind.

In just three weeks, 70 percent of those on oral medication were able to stop taking their medicine altogether; 36 percent of the insulin-takers were able to discontinue the drug. Others in the study were able to reduce their medication requirement. In a Harvard study of 91,000 women, averaging 10 grams daily of cereal fiber lowered the risk of type 2 diabetes by 36 percent. The practical lesson is clear: Add more fiber to your diet and stay active.

Food	Serving Size	Fiber Content (g)
Beans & Legumes		
Beans, kidney, red, canned	½ cup	8
Peas, split, boiled	½ cup	8
Lentils, boiled	½ cup	8
Beans, black, boiled	½ cup	7.5
Beans, pinto, boiled	½ cup	7.5
Refried beans, canned	½ cup	6.5
Lima beans, boiled	½ cup	6.5
Beans, kidney, red, boiled	½ cup	6.5
Beans, baked, canned, plain, or vegetarian	½ cup	6.5
Beans, white, canned	½ cup	6.5
Vegetables (Other)		
Artichokes, boiled	1 cup	9
Peas, boiled	1 cup	9
Vegetable, mixed, boiled	1 cup	8
Lettuce, iceberg	1 head	7.5
Pumpkin, canned	1 cup	7
Peas, canned	1 cup	7
Artichoke, boiled	1 medium	6.5
Brussels sprouts, frozen, boiled	1 cup	6
Parsnips, boiled	1 cup	6
Sauerkraut, canned	1 cup	6
Cereals, Grains, & Pasta		
All-Bran with Extra Fiber (Kellogg's)	½ cup	15
Fiber One (General Mills)	½ cup	14
Granola, homemade	1 cup	13
All-Bran (Kellogg's)	½ cup	9.7
Bulgur wheat, cooked	1 cup	8
Raisin Bran (Kellogg's)	1 cup	8
100% Bran (Post)	⅓ cup	8.3

Bran Chex (Kellogg's)	1 cup	8
Shredded Wheat and Bran	1¼ cups	8
Oat bran, cooked	½ cup	6

Fruits

Avocado, Florida	1 avocado	18
Raspberries, frozen, unsweetened	1 cup	17
Prunes, stewed	1 cup	16
Dates, chopped	1 cup	13
Pears, dried	10 each	13
Avocado, California	1 avocado	8.7
Raspberries, raw	1 cup	8
Blueberries, raw	1 cup	7.6
Papaya, whole	1 fruit	5.5
Figs, dried	2 figs	4.6

Source: Nutrient Data Laboratory. USDA Nutrient Database for Standard Reference. Beltsville, Maryland.

What You Can Do Now

Here are some tips for increasing your fiber intake.

- Read labels. To qualify as a good source of fiber, food should contain at least 2.5 to 3 grams. In addition, the counter in this book can help you find high-fiber foods that fill this bill.
- Make high-fiber substitutions: brown rice for white, whole-grain cereals for processed cereals, bran muffin for a doughnut, bean dips for sour cream dips, black beans or kidney beans for ground beef, and so forth.
- Choose the most nutritious grains—those that have undergone the least processing. Brown rice, for example, is higher in nutrients and fiber, compared to white rice. That's because white rice has been stripped of its husk, germ, and bran layers during processing. Similarly, rolled oats are generally more

nutritious than instant oats. Also, bread made from whole grain has several times the fiber found in white bread.

- Snack on fruits, dried fruits, or raw vegetables, rather than on potato chips or candy.
- Add beans and other legumes to soups and extra beans to chili.
- Purchase packaged cereals that have been fortified with extra fiber.
- Sprinkle your cereal with a few tablespoons of raw wheat bran.
- Eat unpeeled fruit such as apples or pears.

Carbohydrates and the Glycemic Index

Carbohydrates are also classified according to a method called the glycemic index (GI), which was invented in the early 1980s by researchers at the University of Toronto. The glycemic index ranks carbohydrates by the effect they have on your blood sugar (glucose). Foods on the index are rated numerically, with glucose at 100. The higher the number assigned to a food, the faster it converts to glucose. Foods with a rating of 70 or higher are generally considered high glycemic index foods; a rating of 50 to 69, moderate glycemic index foods; and below 50, low glycemic index foods.

High-GI foods, moderate glycemic goods, and low-GI foods yield basically the same amount of food energy (calories), but that is where the similarity ends. If a particular carbohydrate sends your blood sugar soaring, this sets off a reaction that is counterproductive to your efforts. Here is a closer look at exactly what happens: After you eat carbohydrate foods, your body breaks them down into glucose. Some carbohydrates (namely high-GI foods) are dismantled more quickly than others, and this causes a huge spike in your blood glucose. Other carbohydrates (low-GI foods) take longer to break down, and consequently, blood glucose stays relatively even during the digestion process. For combating diabetes, it makes sense to choose mostly low to moderate GI foods, since they help control your blood sugar. This book will show you which carbohydrates fall into these more beneficial GI ranges.

There are many foods that rank so low on the glycemic index that they are really not even rated. This is due to the fact that they have minimal effect on your blood sugar. You can eat as much of them as you like and you don't need to worry about eating them at a certain meal or with another food. These include, but are not limited to, alfalfa sprouts, lettuce, scallions, spinach, tomatoes, peppers, onions, okra, mushrooms, green beans, collards, cucumbers, eggplant, celery, broccoli, and cauliflower. The counter in this book will give you the GI of many foods.

Understanding Glycemic Load (GL)

One issue with the glycemic index is that just because a food ranks high on the index doesn't always mean that a typical serving of it will raise your blood sugar level as rapidly as the index would make it seem. That's where the concept of the glycemic load (GL) comes in. GL takes into account how much carbohydrate is in a real serving size and, based on that, what the food's real potential is to raise blood sugar. This is the formula for computing a food's glycemic load.

The food's GI multiplied by the number of carbohydrate grams being consumed in a given serving divided by 100.

Using this formula, brown rice cakes (which have a high glycemic index of 85), would have a low glycemic load of 12 (85×14 divided by 100). Since the counter includes the GI of many foods, as well as the grams of carbohydrate in specific foods, you can calculate the GL, if you desire, using this formula.

What You Can Do Now

- Use the counter to identify foods that are low and moderate on the glycemic index.
- Choose at least one low-to-moderate GI carbohydrate at each meal.
- Combine proteins and carbohydrates at meals to slow down the rate at which your food is absorbed, as well as the release of blood sugar.
- When you make a high GI choice, balance this with a low GI carbohydrate in the meal or with a lean protein.
- Choose the majority of your carbs from those that have low or no GI ratings. Most vegetables, for example, can be eaten in large amounts, especially salad vegetables. They contain very little carbohydrate and do not raise your blood sugar.
- As a general guideline, fill half of your plate with vegetables such as broccoli, kale, cauliflower and cabbage, and/or other non-starchy vegetables, particularly leafy greens. Fill a quarter of your plate with a serving of starchy carbs that have low to medium GL values (a ½-cup serving is approximately equal to the size of a small clenched fist). The remaining quarter of your plate can be a serving of protein.
- Most fruits (excluding fruit juices, raisins, dried dates, and dried figs) have low GI values. They make great snacks, either by themselves or with low-fat plain yogurt, nut butters, or seed butters.

Food Alert: High-Fructose Corn Syrup

Used as an inexpensive sweetener in many processed foods, high-fructose corn syrup contains a high proportion of glucose, which has been treated with an enzyme that converts part of the glucose to the much sweeter fructose. The major sources of high fructose corn syrup in the diet are soft drinks. Researchers speculate that high-fructose corn syrup may be primarily responsible for the epidemic of obesity and abnormalities seen in a condition called metabolic syndrome, which is a risk factor for type 2 diabetes. Metabolic syndrome is a cluster of symptoms that include insulin resistance, impaired glucose tolerance, abdominal fat, high blood pressure, and elevated cholesterol. The lesson here is to limit your intake of sweetened soft drinks if you are trying to prevent or control diabetes. Read food labels and avoid or reduce foods containing high-fructose corn syrup.

Diabetes-Fighting Proteins

Protein is to your body what a wood frame is to your house, or steel is to a bridge. Nutritionally, it is the most fundamental building material in your body, essential to high-level health because of its role in growth and maintenance. Your body breaks down protein from food into nutrient fragments called amino acids and reshuffles them into new protein to build and rebuild tissue, including muscle. Protein also keeps your immune system functioning up to par, helps carry nutrients throughout the body, has a hand in forming hormones, and is involved in important enzyme reactions such as digestion. When combined with carbohydrates and fat in a meal, protein helps slow your digestion so that glucose is released into your bloodstream more evenly. Protein thus helps control your blood sugar—a role that is supported by research. Studies now confirm that a higher-protein diet promotes improved blood sugar control in people with type 2 diabetes. Generally, a higher protein diet consists of eating 30 percent of your daily calories from protein, 40 percent from carbohydrate, and 30 percent from mostly good fats. If your doctor diagnoses kidney disease, however, you'll want to go on a low-protein diet (10 percent of daily calories from protein), since too much protein can aggravate existing kidney problems. Protein is definitely among the foods that combat diabetes. But it's important to eat the right amount and the right kind of protein to get the health benefits you need. Here is a closer look at the many different forms of protein worth eating if you have diabetes.

What You Can Do Now

- Choose more fish and seafood. Seafood is one of the best anti-diabetes proteins because it's usually low in calories and fat. Fish such as salmon is a little higher in fat, but it is the diabetes-friendly kind: omega-3 fatty acids. One study of people age 40 and older found that those who ate salmon (a fatty fish) every day had a 50 percent lower chance of developing what is termed "glucose intolerance" than those who seldom ate fish. Glucose intolerance simply means that blood glucose has a hard time making its way into cells. Some researchers believe that fatty acids in fish may enhance the delivery of glucose into cells.

- Choose white-meat poultry. An easy, delicious way to enjoy protein is by eating the white meat of poultry. It is lower in fat than dark meat, and low-fat choices are recommended for people with diabetes, mainly to help control weight and stave off heart disease. Poultry skin is loaded with saturated fat, so remove it before cooking.

- Enjoy low-fat dairy products. Not only are dairy foods excellent sources of protein but they also contain valuable calcium. A study of 37,000 women over a 10-year period found that a diet high in low-fat dairy products lowered the risk of type 2 diabetes in middle age. Researchers believe that calcium may promote normal insulin action. Choose skim or low-fat dairy to help keep your blood sugar in line. Calcium, of course, keeps bones and teeth strong, and may even enhance weight loss.

- Eggs are okay. There is good news for egg lovers: yes, you can enjoy eggs, even up to one a day. Eggs are one of the least expensive forms of protein you can choose. Consider trying a special brand of eggs that are high in omega-3 fats, the healthy fat that helps prevent and control diabetes.
- Learn to love beans and legumes. These foods are vegetarian proteins with abundant nutrition, including lots of fiber. Fiber in foods helps keep blood sugar in line. One-half cup of beans contains as much protein as 3 ounces of broiled steak or chicken breast.
- Keep beef choices lean. Although fatty red meat has been linked to a higher risk of diabetes, you do not have to forgo it altogether. Simply opt for those with the word *loin* or *round* in the name, like *sirloin* and eye of the *round*. Trimming excess fat before cooking reduces fat up to 50 percent, and added fat can be kept to a minimum by using low-fat cooking methods, such as broiling, grilling and roasting, or moist-heat cooking methods such as braising and stewing. Incidentally, lean beef has only one more gram of saturated fat than a skinless chicken breast. Lean beef is also an excellent source of zinc, iron, and vitamin B12.
- A great meat choice is pork tenderloin. Pork used to have a bad reputation as a fattening meat. Not anymore. This tasty and versatile white meat is 31 percent leaner than 20 years ago, and worth putting on your menu.
- Soy is a near-perfect diabetic food, well researched in people with diabetes, with compelling findings. Soy improves kidney function in type 1 and type 2 diabetes, reduces abnormally high cholesterol, improves blood flow through arteries, and reduces insulin resistance. This is a condition in which the body does not respond to glucose properly and is seen most commonly in type 2 diabetes. Insulin resistance is a

major risk factor for type 2 diabetes. Thus, introducing more soy into your diet is an important move. Just 25 grams of soy protein daily can help lower cholesterol and reduce the risk of heart disease, which is the leading complication among people with uncontrolled diabetes. Here are some ways to slip soy into your diet.

- Use soy milk on your cereal and blended into smoothies.
- Try soy burgers in place of hamburgers.
- Use textured soy protein in recipes calling for ground beef.
- Snack on soy-based nutrition bars, rather than on candy bars.
- Use tofu on crackers and rice cakes, and in Italian recipes like lasagna to replace all or part of the ricotta cheese. Tofu can also be blended into shakes and smoothies, plus used as a base for dips.
- Munch on soy nuts or soy chips, available at most health food stores.
- Bake using soy flour to replace some of the flour in recipes.

- Try "protein to go." Many different types of meal replacements, such as shakes and bars, have been formulated expressly for people with diabetes. They're worth checking into and make great snacks or full meals when combined with fruit or vegetables. Generally, these products are made with unique blends of slowly digested carbohydrates. "Slowly digested" means that sugar is not immediately broken down and absorbed into the blood, which helps avoid peaks in blood sugar. Consistently maintaining optimal blood sugar levels over time can help reduce the complications of diabetes. Check the label to be sure the product contains at least 6 grams of protein, and is low in sugar and fat.

Food Alert: Red Meat

A study that took place over an 8-year period at the Brigham and Women's Hospital and Harvard Medical School has shown that women who eat five or more servings of red meat on a weekly basis have an increased risk of developing type 2 diabetes. The 37,309 women were part of the Women's Health Study, which was designed by Brigham and Women's Hospital primarily to evaluate the risks and benefits of low-dose aspirin and vitamin E in the prevention of cardiovascular disease (CVD) and cancer. The participants were aged 45 and up, and did not originally have histories of CVD, cancer, or type 2 diabetes. Red meat was defined as beef, hamburger, lamb, and pork, and red processed meat as hot dogs, bacon, sausage, salami, and bologna. The women who ate the five or more servings of red meat weekly were 29 percent more likely to develop type 2 diabetes. Those who ate processed red meat five or more times weekly fared worse: they were 43 percent more likely to develop type 2 diabetes than women who ate only one serving weekly. The study was published in the September 2004 issue of *Diabetes Care*.

Diabetes-Fighting Fats

Dietary fat, a necessary nutrient and an energy source for the body, has been linked to the development of insulin resistance in both animals and humans when eaten in excess. Many studies suggest that higher levels of total fat in the diet result in greater insulin resistance. In addition, it appears that different types of fat have different effects on insulin action. Saturated fats—the kind found in animal fats and butter—have been implicated in causing insulin resistance, whereas unsaturated fats (which come from vegetables and fish) do not appear to have adverse effects on insulin action. Thus, as with carbohydrates and protein, it is important to choose the right types of fat, because clearly not all fats are created equal.

Oils such as safflower oil, sunflower oil, corn oil, soybean oil, and cottonseed oil are polyunsaturated fats. Already mentioned is a special group of polyunsaturated fats known as the omega-3 fatty acids, which are abundant in fish, and are now considered essential fats that must be included in your diet. People with type 2 diabetes sometimes have higher levels of triglycerides and cholesterol than do people without the disease because the liver more readily converts carbohydrates into fats (including triglycerides). Omega-3 fatty acids appear to counteract this conversion and thus may have a beneficial effect on triglyceride levels.

Monounsaturated fats have a protective effect on blood cholesterol levels. They help lower the bad cholesterol, but maintain higher levels of the good cholesterol. They also help keep blood pressure in check and reduce levels of triglycerides in the blood. Monounsaturated fats are plentiful in olive oil, canola oil, and peanut oil, and in fish from cold waters, such as salmon, mackerel, halibut, swordfish, black cod, and rainbow trout, and in shellfish.

As for other dietary fats, watch out for foods containing *trans-fatty acids*. These are produced when vegetable oils are altered chemically through a process called hydrogenation, in which hydrogen is forced into the oil to make it more solid and more spreadable at room temperature. Some margarines and numerous processed foods such as fast foods, snacks, and baked goods are high in trans-fatty acids. These commercially processed unsaturated fats behave more like saturated fats.

Research indicates that hydrogenated fats and the trans-fatty acids they contain may elevate LDL cholesterol and lower beneficial HDL cholesterol. The counter in this book can help you identify foods that are free of trans fats.

FOODS HIGH IN HEALTHY FATS

Best Sources of Monounsaturated Fats	*Best Sources of Polyunsaturated Fats*
Nuts: all types	Walnuts
Herring, Atlantic, pickled	Sunflower seeds
Olive oil	Sunflower oil
Canola oil	Soybeans
Salmon	Vegetable oil
Peanut oil	Sesame oil
Soybeans	Pumpkin seeds
Avocado	Soybean oil
Sesame seeds	Corn oil

What You Can Do Now

- Stick to low-fat and non-fat food choices: lean proteins like white-meat poultry, fish, and egg whites; low-fat dairy products; low-fat salad dressings; and other reduced-fat foods.
- Cut the fat from your diet by making healthful substitutions. For example: a baked potato for French fries; low-fat milk for whole milk; plain yogurt for sour cream or mayonnaise; ice milk or frozen yogurt for ice cream; a grilled chicken sandwich for a cheeseburger; fat-free pretzels for potato chips, to name just a few lower-fat substitutions.
- Broil, bake, or microwave foods, rather than frying them.
- Remove skin from chicken prior to cooking.
- Watch out for "hidden" fat in certain foods too. Fat

is added to crackers, cookies, breads, and rolls. You may not see it, but it's there.

- Read food labels. Even foods claiming to be low fat or natural may contain trans fats. That being so, avoid food products that have the words "hydrogenated" or "partially hydrogenated" on their labels. Hydrogenated fats are trans fats. Look for products that say "trans free" or "0 grams trans fat."
- Limit or avoid using stick margarine, which is the most highly hydrogenated fat of all. Softer tub and liquid margarines are lower in trans fats and are a better alternative. Or, check out the new "trans-free" margarines made without trans fats.
- Avoid cooking with stick margarine or shortening. Substitute vegetable oil. Or, for a fat-free recipe, replace the fat with applesauce or fruit puree.
- Choose margarines and other fats that contain liquid vegetable oil as the first ingredient and no more than two grams of saturated fat per tablespoon.
- Cut back on foods that are fried in vegetable shortening, such as French fries or fried chicken.
- Use olive oil in place of margarine—for dipping breads, rolls, or whole-wheat bagels.
- Use olive oil or canola oil to sauté vegetables and other foods.

Colorful Fruits and Vegetables

The most colorful foods on earth—apricots, mangoes, strawberries, carrots, sweet potatoes, red bell peppers, tomatoes, broccoli, and so forth—are among the best foods that combat diabetes because they are brimming with plant pigments called "carotenoids." These nutrients are useful in preventing diabetic complications.

The most well known of the carotenoids is beta carotene, which gives carrots and other vegetables their characteristic orange color. Once ingested, beta-carotene is converted to vitamin A in the body on an as-needed basis. As an antioxidant, beta carotene's main role is to detoxify tissue-damaging free radicals. This amazing nutrient can also destroy free radicals after they're formed. Other important carotenoids include alpha carotene, cryptoxanthin, gamma carotene, lutein, and lycopene—all found mostly in fruits and vegetables.

Evidence has cropped up that people with diabetes (type 1 and type 2) have low levels of these protective nutrients in their bodies. With carotenoids in short supply, you could be putting yourself in harm's way of developing diabetic complications. Thus, increasing your fruit and vegetable consumption may be therapeutic if you have diabetes. Not only that, these substances may protect against diabetes. In a study of overweight women, a single daily serving of carrots, yams, or sweet potatoes cut the risk of type 2 diabetes by 27 percent, and 1½ servings of spinach or kale cut the risk by 14 percent.

What You Can Do Now

Here are some tips for super-charging your diet with carotenoids.

- Colorize your plate with as many colorful vegetables as you can. The more colorful your food selections, the more carotenoids you'll eat.
- Eat canned soups with a tomato base.
- Drink vegetable juices rather than sodas.
- Eat a hefty serving of tomatoes or tomato-based foods at least twice a week or more.
- Add extra tomato sauce or paste to soups or stews.
- Eat sandwiches and salads with tomatoes.
- Make sure fruits and vegetables are as fresh as possible. Once they're plucked from the vine or harvested from the ground, their antioxidant power starts to dwindle.
- Snack on raw fruits and vegetables to get the most

carotenoids. One exception, though, is carrots, which actually release more carotenoids when cooked.
- Enjoy exotic fruits such as guavas or mangoes for a change of pace.
- Blend cooked carrots or pumpkin into a smoothie.

High Vitamin C Foods

Also known as ascorbic acid, vitamin C is a water-soluble nutrient that can be synthesized by many animals, but not by humans. Plentiful in citrus fruits, melons, tomatoes, and dark green vegetables, it is an essential nutrient in our diets and functions primarily in the formation of connective tissues such as collagen. Vitamin C is also involved in immunity and cholesterol reduction. As an antioxidant, vitamin C keeps free radicals from destroying the outermost layers of cells. Vitamin C also manufactures collagen, which is helpful for bleeding gums and slow wound-healing, both of which can occur with diabetes.

If you have diabetes, you require more vitamin C. Here's why: Insulin helps ferry vitamin C into cells, but excessive levels of blood glucose inhibit this process. Consequently, many diabetics have low levels of vitamin C in their cells. In fact, many studies show that people with diabetes have bodily concentrations of vitamin C that are at least 30 percent lower than people without the disease. If this deficiency becomes chronic and goes uncorrected, you're putting yourself in harm's way of conditions that can further aggravate your health.

TEN TOP FOOD SOURCES OF VITAMIN C		
Food	*Serving Size*	*Vitamin C Content (mg)*
Acerola cherry juice	1 cup	3,872
Acerola cherries, raw	1 cup	1,644

Currants, black	1 cup	456
Peppers, sweet, yellow, raw	1 pepper	341
Peaches, frozen, sliced, unsweetened	1 cup	236
Peppers, sweet, red, raw	1 pepper	226
Papaya	1 fruit	188
Guava	1 fruit	165
Chili peppers, green or red, raw	1 pepper	109
Peppers, sweet, green, raw	1 pepper	106

Source: Nutrient Data Laboratory. USDA Nutrient Database for Standard Reference. Beltsville, Maryland.

What You Can Do Now

- Eat at least one citrus fruit daily.
- Take in extra vitamin C by drinking citrus juice rather than sodas.
- Eat fresh sources of vitamin C whenever possible. Cooking destroys much of the vitamin C in foods.
- Be aware that certain substances inhibit the absorption of vitamin C. These include alcohol, oral contraceptives, smoking, and tetracycline. If using any of these substances, increase your intake of vitamin C–rich foods.

Fruits and Vegetables in General

The evidence is convincing: Eat more fruits and vegetables and you slash your risk of type 2 diabetes and reverse its course if you have it. Proof of this comes from decades of studies showing that vegetarians have lower rates of diabetes and more chronic degenerative diseases than non-vegetarians, for that matter. Vegetarians are less likely to die from heart disease (a threat to diabetics), and vegetarian diets low in saturated fat can actually help reverse severe coronary artery disease. Vegetarians also have a lower incidence of high blood pressure (which is a risk factor for kidney disease in diabetics), independent of body weight and sodium intake. The reason that the vegetarian diet is so protective against diabetes and its complications is largely because a plant-based diet is lower in saturated fat, cholesterol, and animal protein and higher in fiber, phytochemicals, antioxidants, and other diabetes-fighting nutrients. You can eat like a vegetarian without actually being one. Here's how.

What You Can Do Now

- Season your foods with chopped garlic or onion. Both foods are thought to help control blood sugar.
- Eat a salad every day.
- Eat a variety of fruits and vegetables.
- Try a new fruit or vegetable every week.
- Include at least two vegetables with lunch and dinner.
- Double your portion of vegetables at lunch or dinner.
- Top your breakfast cereal with fresh berries.
- Eat baked potatoes topped with broccoli.
- Add extra vegetables to soups and stews.
- Prepare vegetable or fruit platters to take to parties.
- When eating out, order sandwiches prepared with tomato and lettuce.
- Go meatless several times a week.
- At restaurants, choose vegetarian selections or international dishes.
- Eat vegetable burgers, rather than hamburgers, more frequently.
- For pizza, order one topped with vegetables rather than one with meat.
- Snack on fresh fruits and raw vegetables.
- Choose more non-meat sources of protein, such as

beans and dairy products, all of which can provide plenty of protein.

• Add seitan, a meat substitute made from wheat gluten and which has a meat-like consistency, to your favorite bean chili recipe.

• Spread hummus (pureed garbanzo beans) on cucumber slices or use it as sandwich spread instead of mayonnaise.

• Look to vegetable sources for additional calcium. One serving of tofu or a cup of most greens, like spinach, has nearly as much calcium as a glass of whole milk. Sesame seeds, broccoli, and sea vegetables are good sources of calcium, and many vegetarian foods like orange juice and soy milk are now calcium fortified.

• Combine a vegetarian protein called "textured vegetable protein" with tomato sauce, onions, beans, and seasoning for a spicy chili, or use it as a base for veggie burgers.

• Try burgers, franks, and sausages that are made from soy, egg, or wheat protein.

• Add soy pepperoni to veggie pizza, or combine sliced soy sausage with peppers, onions, and potatoes for a hearty stir-fry.

High Niacin (Vitamin B3) Foods

B vitamins are involved in the metabolism of carbohydrate, fat, and protein and are essential for the health of the nervous system, skin, and digestive system. Some compelling evidence shows that niacin may prevent the development of diabetes. Good sources of niacin include beef liver, enriched and whole-grain cereals, and fish.

TEN TOP FOOD SOURCES OF NIACIN

Food	Serving Size	Niacin Content (mg)
General Mills Total	¾ cup	26
Various other ready-to-eat cereals (Raisin Bran, Corn Flakes, Product 19, Wheat Bran Flakes)	¾ cup–1 cup	20
Beef liver	3 oz	15
Chicken breast	½ breast	15
Fish, tuna salad	1 cup	14
Fish, swordfish	1 piece	13
Fast food submarine sandwich, tuna salad	6" sub	11
Fish, halibut	½ fillet	11
Fish, tuna, light, canned in water	3 oz	11
Duck	½ duck	11

Source: Nutrient Data Laboratory. USDA Nutrient Database for Standard Reference. Beltsville, Maryland.

What You Can Do Now

- Enjoy niacin-rich cereals for breakfast through the week.
- Prepare salads using the darkest-leaf lettuce possible (like Romaine). These varieties are higher in nutrients.
- Look for ways to incorporate spinach and other green leafy vegetables into recipes such as those for muffins, soups, lasagna, and casseroles.
- Try to eat 2 to 3 fish meals weekly.

High Biotin Foods

Biotin is a B vitamin involved in metabolism, helping your body make and use fats and amino acids. It steps up the activity of an enzyme called glucokinase, which is responsible for helping your liver utilize glucose. In diabetes, glucokinase concentrations are in short supply. Good sources of biotin include liver, mushrooms, egg yolks, and strawberries.

TEN TOP FOOD SOURCES OF BIOTIN

Food	Serving Size	Biotin Content (mcg)
Chicken liver	3 oz	138
Beef liver	3 oz	30
Egg, whole	1 large	10
Mushrooms, canned	1 cup	5
Egg yolk	1 large	4
Salmon, canned	3 oz	4
Pork chop	3 oz ·	4
Strawberries	1 cup	3
Banana pudding	1 serving	3
Broccoli, fresh	1 cup	2

Source: Nutrient Data Laboratory. USDA Nutrient Database for Standard Reference. Beltsville, Maryland.

What You Can Do Now
- Sprinkle wheat germ on yogurt or cereal.
- Enjoy salads made with dark leafy vegetables.
- Have whole eggs several times a week.

High Vitamin B6 Foods
Vitamin B6 (pyroxidine) is a rather amazing nutrient because it influences nearly every system in the body. For example, it assists in creating amino acids, turning carbohydrates into glucose, metabolizing fats, producing neurotransmitters (chemicals which relay nerve impulses), and manufacturing antibodies to ward off infection. Also, vitamin B6 is needed to prevent the buildup of homocysteine in the blood, a toxic by-product of the amino acid methionine that can eventually lead to atherosclerosis

(hardening of the arteries). For all these reasons, foods containing this nutrient are important in a diet to combat diabetes and its complications. Excellent sources are listed in the table below.

TEN TOP FOOD SOURCES OF VITAMIN B6		
Food	**Serving Size**	**Vitamin B6 Content (mg)**
Various ready-to-eat cereals (All Bran, Total, Product 19, Wheat Bran Flakes, Corn Flakes, Special K)	¾ cup	2–3
Fish, tuna, yellow fin	3 oz	1
Beef	3 oz	1
Turkey	3 oz	1
Chestnuts	1 cup	.7
Fish, halibut	½ fillet	.6
Potato, baked with skin	1 large	.6
Prune juice, canned	1 cup	.6
Duck	½ duck	.5
Banana	1 raw	.5

Source: Nutrient Data Laboratory. USDA Nutrient Database for Standard Reference. Beltsville, Maryland.

What You Can Do Now

- Enjoy vitamin B6–rich cereals for breakfast through the week.
- Stuff avocadoes with tuna, chicken, or shrimp salad.
- Peel and freeze ripe bananas (before they spoil) and use them in smoothies for an ice-cream–like treat.
- Have a cup or half-cup of prune juice before going to bed at night. It has an overnight cleansing effect on your digestive system, besides being a great source of vitamin B6.

High Vitamin B12 Foods

Vitamin B12 also regulates a host of functions in the body. Among the most vital is the production of red blood cells. Vitamin B12 is the director in this process, making sure that enough cells are manufactured. Without vitamin B12, red blood cell production falls off, and the result is misshapen cells and anemia. A deficiency of this B vitamin can cause numbness of the feet, a problem to which diabetics are prone. The best sources of this nutrient are listed below.

TEN TOP FOOD SOURCES OF VITAMIN B12

Food	Serving Size	Vitamin B12 Content (mcg)
Clams	3 oz	84
Beef liver	3 oz	71
Turkey	1 cup	48
Chicken	1 cup	14
Oysters	3 oz	13
Clam chowder	1 cup	10
Alaska King crab	3 oz	10
Salmon	½ fillet	9
Sardines	3 oz.	10
General Mills Whole Grain Total	¾ cup	6.5

Source: Nutrient Data Laboratory. USDA Nutrient Database for Standard Reference. Beltsville, Maryland.

What You Can Do Now

- Enjoy shellfish for dinner on occasion, especially when dining out.
- Serve sardines on whole-wheat crackers for an appetizing snack.
- Stick to lean proteins like chicken and turkey for entrees.
- Try a filling lunch of clam chowder with a side salad.

High Magnesium Foods

Magnesium is the maestro of more than 400 metabolic reactions in your body. Some examples: It helps orchestrate the protein-making machinery inside the cells of soft tissues; helps direct the metabolism of potassium, calcium, and vitamin D; is necessary for the release of energy; helps your muscles relax after contracting; is involved in glucose metabolism; and plays a central role in the secretion and action of insulin.

Diabetes experts have known for some time that people with type 1 and type 2 diabetes are often deficient in magnesium. This deficiency is most likely related to increased losses of urinary magnesium as a result of chronic glycosuria (glucose in the urine).

In people with type 2 diabetes, magnesium deficiency makes the body's cells less sensitive to insulin, according to a number of studies. Severe magnesium deficiency can cause abnormalities in the function of the heart and is possibly related to cardiovascular disease, heart attack, and high blood pressure.

TEN TOP FOOD SOURCES OF MAGNESIUM

Food	Serving Size	Magnesium Content (mg)
Fish, halibut	½ fillet	170
Spinach, canned	1 cup	163
Bulgur wheat, dry	½ cup	115
Oat bran, raw	½ cup	110
Barley, pearl, raw	½ cup	79
Cornmeal, whole grain, yellow	½ cup	77
Soybeans, boiled	½ cup	74
Snacks, trail mix, tropical	½ cup	67
Beans, black, boiled	½ cup	60
Kellogg's All Bran Original	½ cup	54

Source: Nutrient Data Laboratory. USDA Nutrient Database for Standard Reference. Beltsville, Maryland.

What You Can Do Now
- Select fewer refined grains and choose whole grains like oats or barley instead.
- Enjoy guacamole with whole-grain crackers.
- Have sandwiches prepared with whole-grain breads.
- Opt for more legumes and leafy vegetables in your diet.
- Snack on fruits like apples, apricots, and cantaloupe, which are also high in magnesium.

Honorable Mention Foods and Beverages

Nuts

Eating a handful of nuts or a tablespoon of peanut butter five times a week may reduce your risk of adult-onset diabetes by more than 20 percent, according to a report in the *Journal of the American Medical Association*. While nuts do contain some saturated fat, they are high in unsaturated fat and other nutrients, such as fiber and magnesium, which help balance glucose and insulin levels and control cholesterol levels. If you like peanut butter, read labels, since some brands are high in sugar. Nuts and peanut butter are high in calories too, so if you decide to munch on them regularly, do so as a replacement for consumption for processed carbohydrates or red or processed meats.

What You Can Do Now
- Sprinkle nuts over yogurt or cereals.
- Coat fish with ground nutmeats and bake.
- Spread peanut butter on celery for snacks.
- Put a tablespoon of peanut butter in vanilla, chocolate, or banana smoothies.

Tea and Coffee

Drinking coffee (1 to 2 cups a day) is associated with a reduced risk for type 2 diabetes, according to some recent research. Supposedly, there are compounds in coffee that help the body metabolize sugar. Also, more and more studies are finding that the antioxidants in tea, both green and black, are powerful weapons when it comes to fighting diabetes. They seem to improve insulin activity. One study, for example, of 17,413 persons who were 40 to 65 years of age and were tea or coffee drinkers had a reduced risk for type 2 diabetes. This is great news for coffee and tea drinkers, but if you're not among them, don't change your beverage choices on the basis of these findings. Drinking an excess of caffeinated beverages has been linked to heart risks, rheumatoid arthritis, and other ailments. It can also increase sleeplessness and affect heart rhythm.

What You Can Do Now
- If you're a coffee drinker, continue to enjoy your java, but stay within moderate amounts (1 to 2 cups a day).
- Consider adding tea to your menus as a beverage.
- Try making iced green tea as a refreshing summertime beverage.

Alcohol
It's perfectly okay to enjoy a few drinks through the week without jeopardizing your blood sugar control. In men and women, moderate alcohol consumption is associated with about a 30 percent reduction in the risk of type 2 diabetes. In a 10-year Harvard University study, which involved 109,690 women ages 25 to 42 years, researchers found that women who had about half a drink to two drinks a day were 58 percent less likely than nondrinkers to develop type 2 diabetes. But those who had more than two drinks of hard liquor a day faced more than double the risk of nondrinkers. Previous studies in men have also linked heavy drinking with an increased diabetes risk.

What You Can Do Now

- Make sure your alcohol intake stays within reasonable limits. The American Diabetes Association recommends that daily intake of alcohol be limited to a moderate amount: one drink per day or less for adult women and two drinks per day or less for adult men.
- If you don't drink, don't take it up now. Alcohol can be addictive and has adverse health effects on organs if used in excess.
- When enjoying a cocktail, have it with a meal and not on an empty stomach, or else you could cause swings in your blood sugar.

There you have it—an overview of foods that truly combat diabetes. Clearly, food is one of the chief tools you can use to prevent diabetes, control it, and stay healthy. It helps keep your blood sugar in line, provides energy for exercise and daily activities, and supplies the nutrients needed for health and healing. Food is nourishment and medicine all rolled into one. Now let's look at how to leverage this information into a diet you'll enjoy—and your body will love.

CHAPTER 2

A SIX-STEP DIET TO COMBAT DIABETES

There really is no single "diabetic diet" anymore. That's good news, and it means you have a lot of leeway when choosing foods to eat each day. Even so, you'll want to stay within certain broad guidelines to make sure your nutritional choices are working to prevent or control diabetes. In its 2007 "Clinical Practice Guidelines," the American Diabetes Association gives the following important parameters.

- Consume 45 to 65 percent of your total daily calories from carbohydrates; 20 to 35 percent of calories from fat; and 10 to 35 percent from protein. The diet planning guidelines in this chapter and the next will show you how to do this.
- Saturated fat intake should be less than 7 percent of your total daily calories, and your intake of trans fat should be minimized.
- Keep track of your carbohydrate intake because carbs have the most impact on your blood sugar. In

other words, the amount of carbohydrates you eat (rather than fats or proteins) will determine how high your blood sugar levels rise. All carbohydrates will raise your blood sugar to a similar degree. In general, 1 gram of carbohydrates raises blood sugar by 3 points in people who weigh 200 pounds, 4 points for weights of 150 pounds, and 5 points for 100 pounds.

- If you already have diabetes, using the glycemic index of foods to guide food selection may provide a modest additional benefit for blood sugar control. The counter can help you in this regard.

- Choose foods that are high in fiber whenever possible, since they help control blood sugar.

- For weight loss, it is better to cut your calorie intake and increase your physical activity. Losing weight will help you overcome insulin resistance and reduce your risk of developing type 2 diabetes. Low-carbohydrate diets (restricting total carbohydrate to less than 130 grams a day) are not recommended if you are overweight. The long-term effects of these diets are unknown, and although such diets produce short-term weight loss, keeping the weight off is difficult, and the impact of these diets on heart health is uncertain.

- Feel free to eat artificial sweeteners. They are safe when consumed within the acceptable daily intake levels established by the Food and Drug Administration (FDA).

- If you have prediabetes or diabetes, consider getting individualized nutrition help from a registered dietitian familiar with the components of diabetes management. This form of nutrition, termed *medical nutrition therapy*, should be covered by insurance and other payors.

How to Plan Your Diet in 6 Easy Steps

This diet plan incorporates six different food groups with recommended servings in each group: starchy carbohydrates, non-starchy vegetables, fruit, low-fat dairy products, lean proteins, fats, sweets, and miscellaneous foods. With this plan, you get variety, plenty of choices, and lots of flavor. Here is a step-by-step guide to planning your diet according to these food groups.

Step One: Eat at least 6 Servings a Day from Starchy Carbohydrates

This food group includes bread, cereal, rice, and pasta. These foods contain mostly carbohydrates and are high in fiber. Grains such as wheat, rye, and oats belong to this group. So do starchy vegetables like potatoes, peas, beans, legumes, and corn. Typical serving sizes are as follows.

1 slice of bread
2 slices reduced calorie bread
½ of a medium bagel (1 ounce)
½ an English muffin or pita bread
1 6-inch tortilla
¾ cup dry (ready-to-eat) cereal
½ cup cooked cereal
1 medium potato, sweet potato, or yam
½ cup potato, yam, peas, corn, or cooked beans
½ cup winter squash
½ cup cooked rice or pasta

Step Two: Eat 3 to 5 Servings of Vegetables Daily

Non-starchy vegetables occupy the second food group. All of these vegetables are naturally low in fat and good choices to include often in your meals or have them as a low-calorie snack. Vegetables are full of vitamins, minerals, antioxidants, phytochemicals, and fiber. This group includes spinach, chicory, sorrel, Swiss chard, broccoli, cabbage, bok choy, Brussels sprouts, cauliflower, kale, carrots, tomatoes, cucumbers, and lettuce. (Starchy vegetables such as potatoes, corn, peas, and lima beans are considered starchy carbohydrates.) A typical serving is as follows.

1 cup raw
½ cup cooked
1 cup vegetable juice

Tips for Buying Vegetables

- Look for fresh produce that is crisp and not wilted. Fresh equates with nutritious.
- Avoid buying too much precut produce. Cutting exposes more surface area to oxygen, which breaks down and destroys nutrients.
- When purchasing a salad mix, look for a colorful medley of greens in the bag. The more color, the more antioxidants, carotenoids, and flavonoids in the salad.
- Always select the brightest, most colorful fruits and vegetables on the shelves. The brighter the color, the more vitamins and other nutrients the produce contains.
- Go for darker shades of green when purchasing lettuce. Dark-leafed vegetables like Romaine lettuce are more rich in folate than are lighter green varieties of lettuce such as iceberg.
- Similarly, buy certain vegetables, such as onions and sweet peppers, in all their various colors, for a greater array of flavonoids.
- For convenience, don't shun canned foods. Although canning can destroy some vitamin C and B vitamins, canned foods still contain considerable nutrition.
- Eat fresh fruits and vegetables within three to four days of purchase; don't let them sit for too long. The longer produce languishes in your refrigerator, the greater the

loss of nutrients. If you can't shop often enough to keep produce fresh, purchase smaller quantities of fruits and vegetables and shop more often. Or, opt for frozen vegetables. They're as high in nutrients as fresh food. Frozen green beans, for example, have more vitamin C than fresh beans stored in the refrigerator for a couple of days. The reason: They were frozen within a few hours of harvesting so, in many cases, their nutritional quality is higher than that of fresh foods. Fresh foods begin to lose nutrients shortly after picking.

- Eat fruits and vegetables raw whenever possible. Generally, raw produce is healthier. In one interesting study, blood levels of vitamins A and E rose significantly in people who ate raw fruits and vegetables for just one week. One exception to the "raw rule": When cooked, carrots yield more carotenoids.

- Limit cutting and dicing of fruits and vegetables in order to prevent their surfaces from overexposure to vitamin-destroying oxygen. As an alternative, cut fruits and vegetables into larger pieces and cover them. Serve as close to mealtime as possible.

- Avoid peeling too. Nutrients and fiber are lost when produce is peeled.

- Don't discard the outer leaves of greens. They contain more nutrients than the inner portions do.

- Make sure the cooking temperature is reached before adding the food. Return the water to boil as quickly as possible after the food has been added.

- Cook foods for the shortest amount of time possible. Use your microwave for quick cooking and for reheating leftovers. Quick cooking methods, at high temperatures with the least exposure to water, preserve the greatest amount of nutrients. By contrast, vitamins in vegetables are easily destroyed with prolonged exposure to heat, water, and air. Other good quick-cooking methods include steaming, stir-frying, and grilling.

- Cook vegetables using a steam basket that fits into a

saucepan. Fill the saucepan with about an inch or two of water. Place vegetables in the basket and cover the saucepan with a tight-fitting lid. Steam vegetables for a few minutes—until tender but still crisp in order to preserve more nutrients.

- In lieu of a steam basket, fill the saucepan with about an inch or less of water. Add vegetables so that they are piled above the water line. Cook for just a few minutes. The point is to reduce contact with water. Water dissolves water-soluble vitamins such as vitamin C and the B vitamins.
- Avoid thawing frozen fruits and vegetables prior to cooking. As foods thaw, microorganisms once dormant in the food begins to multiply, spoiling the food. It's better to cook frozen food without letting it thaw first.
- With a canned food, try to serve its liquid with the food because there are nutrients in the liquid.
- Use any leftover cooking water or canned liquid for soups, sauces, and broths.
- Never overcook vegetables. It destroys vitamin C, which is highly sensitive to heat. In fact, prolonged boiling robs vegetables of 33 to 90 percent of their vitamin C.
- Minimize reheating of food to reduce further nutrient losses.
- Crush or dice garlic prior to cooking in order to liberate its many beneficial cancer-fighting substances.

Step 3: Choose 2 to 4 Servings of Fruit Daily

The next food group is fruits, which also contain carbohydrates. Fruits have plenty of vitamins, minerals, antioxidants, phytochemicals, and fiber. This group includes blackberries, cantaloupe, strawberries, oranges, apples, bananas, peaches, pears, apricots, and grapes. A typical serving is as follows.

½ cup canned fruit
1 small fresh fruit

2 tablespoons of dried fruit
1 cup of melon or raspberries
1 cup of whole strawberries
1 cup fruit juice

Tips for Buying Fruits

- When buying fresh fruits, be on the lookout for bruises on the fruit. Bruising initiates a chemical reaction that causes nutrient content to dwindle.
- Berries are highly perishable. At the store, check for freshness by looking at the bottom of the box. Staining indicates that the fruit has been bruised or is overripe, meaning that it will spoil rapidly and that nutrient loss has already set in.
- Look for a bright red color when purchasing strawberries. Bright color signals exceptional nutritional quality. Avoid berries with too much whiteness at the base; they're less nutritious.
- Sniff fruits such as cantaloupe or berries to test for freshness. A pleasant aroma usually indicates good flavor, ripeness, and nutritional goodness. Fruits such as cantaloupes and mangoes should feel somewhat soft to the touch.

Step 4: Have 2 to 3 Servings a Day of Low-Fat Dairy Products

The third food group contains milk and yogurt—foods that contribute carbohydrates, protein, and some fat to your diet. Choose dairy products that are lower in fat or fat-free; these are also generally lower in calories too. Also, try a variety of lower-fat products, since many brands differ in taste and texture, to find out which one you prefer. Dairy products spoil quickly, so purchase only what you can consume within the next few days. A typical serving is as follows.

1 cup non-fat or low-fat milk
1 cup of yogurt
1 cup non-fat or low-fat buttermilk

Step 5: Enjoy 4 to 6 Ounces Daily of Lean Proteins

This group includes meat, poultry, fish, cheese, tofu, eggs, and peanut butter. Choose from lean meats, poultry, and fish and cut all the visible fat off meat. Keep your portion sizes small. Three ounces is about the size of a deck of cards. You only need 4 to 6 ounces for the whole day, divided between meals. The following serving sizes are equal to 1 ounce of meat, fish, or poultry.

¼ cup cottage cheese
1 egg
1 tablespoon peanut butter
½ cup tofu

Cooking Tips for Protein

- Stick to low-fat cooking methods: grilling, roasting, broiling, steaming, or stewing. These cooking methods also keep meat moist and tasty.
- Marinate meat or poultry prior to grilling it. Marinating helps tenderize meat.
- Be careful not to undercook meat, poultry, or fish, however. Undercooking increases the risk that illness-causing bacteria will form on the food. With meat, for example, cook it to the medium rare or medium stage to be on the safe side. Chicken and fish should be fully cooked.

Step 6: Enjoy Fats, Sweets, and Alcohol in Moderation

Certain foods should be used sparingly in your diet. Foods like potato chips, candy, cookies, cakes, crackers, and fried foods contain a lot of fat or sugar. They aren't as nutritious as vegetables or grains. When selecting fats, make sure to choose monounsaturated or polyunsaturated varieties. Keep your servings small and save them for special treats. A typical serving size includes the following.

1 tablespoon oil
1 tablespoon salad dressing
2 tablespoons low-fat or no-calorie salad dressing
½ cup ice cream
2 small cookies
4 oz glass of wine
12 oz can of beer
1 oz hard liquor

If You Need to Lose Weight

For a diet to be successful, it must be safe, easy to follow, and a cinch to stick to. It must generate results in a reasonable period of time. And, it must help initiate a pattern of healthy habits that lead to lifelong weight control. Happily, the six-step diet plan outlined here can help you accomplish all three.

For starters, it automatically helps you control calories. Despite the popularity of eat-all-you-want diets, calorie reduction remains the preferred way to take off pounds. To lose pounds, you'll need to eat fewer calories each day than you burn off. You can accelerate your weight loss by adding calorie-burning exercise to this equation. Exercise expends additional calories, up to 500 calories an hour, depending on how hard you work out. What's more, bodies that develop more muscle through exercising burn off more calories than do fatter bodies. Under this plan, you'll eat about 1400 to 1600 calories to provide a safe rate of weight loss—about 1 to 2 pounds a week. When you drop pounds at this pace, you're shedding mostly body fat.

This plan is also high in complex carbohydrates.

These foods supply an amazing fat-fighting nutrient— fiber. A growing body of research shows that high fiber eating helps peel off pounds and banish them for good. How exactly does fiber work this weight-loss magic? Mainly by curtailing your food intake. Because fibrous foods provide bulk, you feel full while eating a meal, so you're less tempted to overeat. High-fiber foods also take longer to chew, so your meals last longer. That's a plus, since it takes about 20 minutes after starting a meal for your body to send signals that it's full. And, when eaten with other nutrients like protein, fiber slows the rate of digestion too, curbing your appetite between meals.

Finally, be sure to drink eight to ten glasses of pure water daily. Drinking more water can actually help you stay lean, indirectly. Your kidneys depend on enough water to do their job of filtering waste products from the body. In a water shortage, the kidneys need backup, so they turn to the liver for help. One of the liver's many functions is mobilizing stored fat for energy. By taking on extra assignments from the kidneys, the liver can't do its fat-burning job as well. Fat loss is compromised as a result. You thus have to drink enough water to keep your body's fat-burning processes proceeding full steam ahead.

Reading Food Labels

As you begin to change your diet for the better, make a habit of reading labels on food packages, in addition to using this counter. Required on most foods, the "Nutrition Facts" label is a quick way to get information about serving sizes, calories, fat (including saturated fat and trans fat), cholesterol, sodium, fiber, sugars, carbohydrates, and protein. You'll also find a list of ingredients in descending order by weight. The ingredient list is also a good place to look for healthy ingredients such as soy; monounsaturated fats such as olive, canola, or peanut oils; or whole grains, like whole-wheat flour and oats. By carefully reading nutrition labels, you can make sure you're eating a healthy diet and not getting any surprises.

Some of the most important information is found on the left side of the label and provides total amounts of different nutrients per serving. To make wise choices, pay attention to the following.

Serving Size. The first place to start when you look at the Nutrition Facts label is the serving size and the number of servings in the package. Serving sizes are standardized to make it easier to compare similar foods; they are provided in familiar units, such as cups or pieces, followed by the metric amount, such as the number of grams. The size of the serving on the food package influences the number of calories and all the nutrient amounts listed on the top part of the label. Pay attention to the serving size, especially how many servings there are in the food package.

Calories. The next item to check is the calorie content per serving. If you are trying to lose or maintain your weight, the number of calories you eat counts. You can use labels to compare similar products and determine which contains fewer calories.

Total Fat. Pay close attention to the total fat in food per serving. Total fat includes healthy fats such as mono and polyunsaturated fats, and not-so-healthy fats like saturated and trans fats. Mono and polyunsaturated fats can help to lower your blood cholesterol and protect your heart. Saturated and trans fat can raise your blood cholesterol and increase your risk of heart disease. The cholesterol in food may also increase your blood cholesterol.

Sodium. Sodium does not affect your blood glucose levels. However, many people with diabetes need to watch their sodium intake because an excess can contribute to high blood pressure. If you have high blood pressure, it is a good idea to eat less sodium.

Total Carbohydrate. Look at the grams of total carbohydrate; it includes sugar, complex carbohydrate, and fiber. The grams of sugar and fiber are counted as part of the grams of total carbohydrate. If a food has 5 grams or more fiber in a serving, subtract the fiber grams from the total grams of carbohydrate for a more accurate estimate of the carbohydrate content.

Fiber. Fiber is the part of plant foods that is not digested. The recommendation is to eat 25 to 30 grams of fiber per day. People with diabetes need the same amount of fiber as everyone else.

Sugar Alcohols. Some foods will list sugar alcohols on their labels. Used as artificial sweeteners in many foods, particularly low-carb products, the sugar alcohols include erythritol, sorbitol, maltitol, mannitol, xylitol, lactitol, and isomalt. They are derived from fruit or produced from a sugar called dextrose. Most sugar alcohols contain from .2 to .4 calories per gram (sugar provides 4 calories per gram). Most sugar alcohols are not digested in the small intestine the way regular sugars are. Instead, they pass straight through to the large intestine where they are broken down by fermentation. As a result, they do not raise blood sugar as much as regular sugar does. For this reason, sugar alcohols are thought to be better than sugar for people with diabetes. A downside of sugar alcohols is that, if eaten in excess, they have a laxative effect. The use of sugar alcohols in a product does not necessarily mean the product is low in carbohydrate or calories. And, just because a package says "sugar-free" on the outside, that does not mean that it is calorie- or carbohydrate-free. Always remember to check the label for the grams of carbohydrate and calories.

Percent (%) Daily Value. The percent (%) daily value indicates how much of a specific nutrient one serving of food contains compared to recommendations for the whole day. The percentage is based on a 2,000-calorie diet. If you need more or fewer calories, then your daily values would be different. You can use the percent daily value to check whether a food is high or low in a certain nutrient such as fat or fiber. A product is a *good* source of a particular nutrient if one serving provides 10 to 19 percent of the daily value, *high* in a given nutrient if it contains 20 percent or more of the daily value, and *low* in that nutrient if the daily value is 5 percent or less.

DINING OUT WITH DIABETES

You can find healthy alternatives at just about any restaurant. Here are some tips for making wise choices when dining out, no matter what the cuisine.

Mexican Restaurants

- Ask the wait person for plain, fresh tortillas, instead of fried tortilla chips, to dip in the salsa at your table. Corn tortillas contain less fat than flour ones, but both are good alternatives to fried chips (one 6-inch corn tortilla=1 bread or 1 carbohydrate/starch serving).
- Enjoy the salsa. Load up your tacos, burritos, tortillas, or fajitas with salsa instead of sour cream and high-fat alternatives. Not only is salsa fat-free, but it's also full of vitamins and phytochemicals.
- Ask for regular beans instead of refried beans, which are fried in lard or other types of fat. Not only are beans low in fat, but they are also high in fiber and protein. (1/2 cup boiled beans=1 bread or carbohydrate/starch serving).
- Choose fajitas and build them with vegetables and salsa, rather than with high-fat items such as cheese and sour cream.
- Select bean and rice dishes, which amplify your fiber intake, and spice them up with salsa.

Italian Restaurants

- Enjoy some protein (such as fish, skinless chicken, or lean veal) with a side of vegetables rather than carbohydrate-rich pasta.

- Order meatballs without the pasta.
- Start off with minestrone or gazpacho, vegetable-rich soups that can help reduce your appetite for relatively few calories.
- Ask for dressing on the side and enjoy it in smaller portions. Briefly dip fork in dressing, and then gather salad with fork. This helps you enjoy each bite of salad with a hint of dressing.
- Opt for a red (tomato-based) sauce instead of a white one, which is generally cream- and/or butter-based.
- Try shellfish. Steamed or in a tomato-based broth, mussels, clams, and other shellfish are delicious, low-calorie choices.
- Enjoy veal. Veal is leaner and lower in fat than most beef, especially if you choose a cut that is baked rather than fried.

Asian Restaurants

- Avoid high-fat items, such as deep-fried General Tso's chicken.
- Limit your selection of high-fat meats, such as chicken and duck with skin.
- Most Asian dishes are made with high-sodium soy sauce, so be careful if you must limit sodium intake.
- Use chopsticks. Whether you are a beginner or are experienced, using chopsticks slows down your eating. Chopsticks allow you to eat less by helping you avoid the extra sauce you might get when using a fork or spoon.
- Instead of fried wontons or egg rolls, try the wonton, egg drop, or hot and sour soup.
- Enjoy the vegetables. Sample Asian dishes that may not be staples in your home—baby corn, snap peas, water chestnuts, and sprouts.
- Choose brown rice over white—it's higher in fiber, iron, and zinc.
- Ask for meat or shellfish with vegetables steamed or prepared by stir-frying.
- Choose moo shu dishes, which are generally leaner alternatives.
- Opt for menu items with tofu, miso, or tempeh.

Keeping Track

Using the recommendations above, I've created a work-sheet to help you monitor your weekly intake of foods on this diet plan. The worksheet lists the specific groups of foods you need each day and is organized into one calendar week. Whenever you eat a specific food, simply check off the food in the space provided. This worksheet can serve as a daily reminder of how well you're doing and make diabetic meal planning a breeze.

Day	Starchy carbohydrates	Non-starch vegetables	Fruit	Low-fat dairy	Lean protein	Fats, sweets, alcohol	Water
	6–11 servings	3–5 servings	2–4 servings	2–3 servings	4 to 6 oz daily	Sparingly (Fat–30% or less of daily calories; saturated fat, 7% or less)	8 to 10 cups daily
Sunday	☐☐☐☐ ☐☐☐☐ ☐☐☐	☐☐☐ ☐☐	☐☐ ☐☐	☐☐ ☐	1 oz ☐ 2 oz ☐ 3 oz ☐ 4 oz ☐ 5 oz ☐ 6 oz ☐	Fat: _____ Sweets: _____ Alchohol: _____	☐☐ ☐☐ ☐☐ ☐☐ ☐☐
Monday	☐☐☐☐ ☐☐☐☐ ☐☐☐	☐☐☐ ☐☐	☐☐ ☐☐	☐☐ ☐	1 oz ☐ 2 oz ☐ 3 oz ☐ 4 oz ☐ 5 oz ☐ 6 oz ☐	Fat: _____ Sweets: _____ Alchohol: _____	☐☐ ☐☐ ☐☐ ☐☐ ☐☐

Day	Starchy carbohydrates	Non-starch vegetables	Fruit	Low-fat dairy	Lean protein	Fats, sweets, alcohol	Water
Tuesday	☐☐☐☐ ☐☐☐☐ ☐☐☐	☐☐☐☐ ☐	☐☐	☐☐	1 oz☐ 2 oz☐ 3 oz☐ 4 oz☐ 5 oz☐ 6 oz☐	Fat: _____ Sweets: _____ Alcohol: _____	☐☐ ☐☐ ☐☐ ☐☐ ☐☐
Wednesday	☐☐☐☐ ☐☐☐☐ ☐☐☐	☐☐☐☐ ☐	☐☐	☐☐	1 oz☐ 2 oz☐ 3 oz☐ 4 oz☐ 5 oz☐ 6 oz☐	Fat: _____ Sweets: _____ Alcohol: _____	☐☐ ☐☐ ☐☐ ☐☐ ☐☐

Day	Starchy carbohydrates	Non-starch vegetables	Fruit	Low-fat dairy	Lean protein	Fats, sweets, alcohol	Water
Thursday	☐ ☐ ☐ ☐ ☐ ☐ ☐ ☐ ☐ ☐ ☐	☐ ☐ ☐ ☐ ☐	☐ ☐ ☐ ☐	☐ ☐ ☐	1 oz ☐ 2 oz ☐ 3 oz ☐ 4 oz ☐ 5 oz ☐ 6 oz ☐	Fat: _____ Sweets: _____ Alcohol: _____	☐ ☐ ☐ ☐ ☐ ☐ ☐ ☐ ☐ ☐
Friday	☐ ☐ ☐ ☐ ☐ ☐ ☐ ☐ ☐ ☐ ☐	☐ ☐ ☐ ☐ ☐ ☐	☐ ☐ ☐ ☐	☐ ☐ ☐	1 oz ☐ 2 oz ☐ 3 oz ☐ 4 oz ☐ 5 oz ☐ 6 oz ☐	Fat: _____ Sweets: _____ Alcohol: _____	☐ ☐ ☐ ☐ ☐ ☐ ☐ ☐

Day	Starchy carbohydrates	Non-starch vegetables	Fruit	Low-fat dairy	Lean protein	Fats, sweets, alcohol	Water
Saturday	☐☐☐☐ ☐☐☐☐ ☐☐☐	☐☐☐☐ ☐	☐☐ ☐☐	☐☐ ☐	1 oz ☐ 2 oz ☐ 3 oz ☐ 4 oz ☐ 5 oz ☐ 6 oz ☐	Fat: ____ Sweets: ____ Alcohol: ____	☐☐ ☐☐ ☐☐ ☐☐ ☐☐

CHAPTER 3

A SAMPLE DIABETES-FIGHTING MENU

The following three-day menu shows you what an ideal diet for combating diabetes might look like, based on the information provided in Chapters 1 and 2. This plan uses the principles in the previous chapter: it's high in fiber; balanced with the right kinds of carbohydrates, protein, and fat; and loaded with nutrition. Try these menus and you'll see how easy it is to plan and enjoy this healthful new way of eating. Recipes for items in italics follow this sample menu plan.

Day 1

BREAKFAST
    ½ cup *Low-Fat, Low-Sugar Granola*
    1 cup low-fat milk
    1 slice whole-wheat toast
    1 cup strawberries

MID-MORNING SNACK
    Tropical Freeze

LUNCH
  Tuna Nicoise Salad

MID-AFTERNOON SNACK
  1 cup vegetable juice
  6 whole-wheat crackers

DINNER
  1 serving *Tofu Roll-Ups*
  Tossed green salad with 2 tablespoons *Reduced-Fat
     Blue Cheese Dressing*
  Baked Almond Flan

Nutritional information for day 1: 1,533 calories; 234
grams carbohydrate; 83 grams protein; 24 grams total
fat; 8.5 grams saturated fat; 156 mg cholesterol; 2,722 mg
sodium; 31 grams fiber.

Day 2

BREAKFAST
  1 scrambled egg
  1 whole-wheat English muffin
  ½ grapefruit

MID-MORNING SNACK
  1 cup sugar-free, fat-free fruit yogurt
  1 cup blueberries

LUNCH
  Low-Fat Sloppy Joe, served on a whole-wheat
     hamburger bun
  1 serving *Three-Bean Salad*
  Mocha Smoothie

MID-AFTERNOON SNACK
  Salmon Snacks

DINNER
Barbecued Chicken Breasts
1 cup steamed cauliflower

Nutritional information for day 2: 2,042 calories; 247 grams carbohydrate; 128 grams protein; 53 grams total fat; 12 grams saturated fat; 332 mg cholesterol; 2,596 mg sodium; 27 grams fiber.

Day 3

BREAKFAST
½ bagel spread with reduced-fat cream cheese
1 scrambled egg
1 cup orange juice

MID-MORNING SNACK
1 *Natural Muffin*
1 cup soy milk
1 medium apple

LUNCH
Nut-Crusted Fish Fillets
Rosemary-Sautéed Spinach
⅓ cup *Low-Fat Fried Brown Rice*

MID-AFTERNOON SNACK
Guacamole Dip served with 1 cup raw vegetables

DINNER
1 cup *Low-Fat Creamy Asparagus Soup*
Shrimp Scampi with Broccoli
Tossed Salad (greens with assorted salad vegetables) with nonfat salad dressing
Quick Sugar-Free Cherry Cobbler

Nutritional information for day 3: 1,366 calories; 163 grams carbohydrate; 53 grams protein; 48 grams total fat; 4 grams saturated fat; 336 mg cholesterol; 1,569 mg sodium; 27 grams fiber.

The Recipes

GUACAMOLE DIP

1 cup ripe mashed avocado (2 avocados)
1 tablespoon grated onion
1 tablespoon lemon juice
½ teaspoon salt
¼ teaspoon chili powder
⅓ cup reduced-fat mayonnaise

1. Combine all ingredients except mayonnaise and mix well.
2. Place mixture in a bowl and spread mayonnaise over the top, sealing the edges with plastic wrap. Chill.
3. When ready to serve, blend mayonnaise into avocado mixture. Serve with cut-up fresh vegetables instead of chips.

Makes 6 servings.

Nutritional information per serving: 104 calories; 4 grams carbohydrate; 0 grams protein; 10 grams total fat; 1 gram saturated fat; 0 mg cholesterol; 98 mg sodium; 2 grams fiber.

SALMON SNACKS

1 15-oz can salmon
1 8-oz package nonfat cream cheese
1 teaspoon dried dill
2 tablespoons onion, minced
6 whole-wheat or low-carb tortillas

1. Drain canned salmon and remove bones.

2. In a small bowl, combine salmon, cream cheese, dill, and onion. Mix well.

3. Spread about 2 tablespoons of the mixture over each tortilla. Roll up each tortilla tightly. Wrap each one with clear plastic wrap and chill for 2 to 3 hours.

4. Slice each tortilla into bite-sized pieces.

Makes about 36 appetizers.

Nutritional information per appetizer: 33 calories; 4 grams carbohydrate; 4 grams protein; 1 gram total fat; 0 grams saturated fat; 5 mg cholesterol; 122 mg sodium; 0 grams fiber.

TROPICAL FREEZE

½ cup unsweetened pineapple juice
½ banana
¼ cup instant fat-free dry milk
½ teaspoon coconut extract
1 cup crushed ice

1. Place ingredients in the blender jar in the order listed. Cover blender jar.

2. Process on liquify until smooth. Serve immediately.

Makes 1 serving.

Nutritional information per serving: 185 calories; 37 grams carbohydrate; 8 grams protein; 0 grams total fat; 0 grams saturated fat; 0 mg cholesterol; 93 mg sodium; 1 gram fiber.

MOCHA SMOOTHIE

1 teaspoon instant coffee crystals
1 tablespoon hot water

½ cup low-fat milk or soy milk
2 small scoops sugar-free fat-free vanilla ice cream
1 tablespoon sugar-free chocolate syrup

1. Dissolve coffee crystals in hot water and place in blender jar.
2. Add remaining ingredients in the order listed.
3. Cover blender jar and process on puree until smooth. Serve immediately.

Makes 1 serving.

Nutritional information per serving: 184 calories; 37 grams carbohydrate; 8 grams protein; 1 gram total fat; 0 grams saturated fat; 5 mg cholesterol; 152 mg sodium; 1 gram fiber.

LOW-FAT, LOW-SUGAR GRANOLA

2½ cups apple juice
½ cup reduced-calorie syrup (fructose-sweetened)
2 teaspoon vanilla
14 cups rolled oats
1 package dried apricots, cut in pieces
2 tablespoons cinnamon
2 teaspoons nutmeg
Vegetable oil cooking spray

1. In a large saucepan, heat apple juice, syrup, and vanilla to boiling, then remove from heat. Stir in oats and apricots and moisten thoroughly. Mix in cinnamon and nutmeg.
2. Spray three cookie sheets with vegetable oil spray. Spread oat mixture onto the sheets and spray the mixture with vegetable oil spray three times to coat it.
3. Bake in a 325° oven until dry and crisp—about 50

minutes. Stir the mixture frequently during baking. Remove from oven. Let cool and pack in airtight containers. The granola does not need refrigeration.

Makes 28 one-half cup servings.

Nutritional information per serving: 184 calories; 34 grams carbohydrate; 7 grams protein; 0 grams total fat; 0 grams saturated fat; 0 mg cholesterol; 11 mg sodium; 5 grams fiber.

NATURAL MUFFINS

1 cup oatmeal flour (blend rolled oats in a blender
until fine)
1 cup cornmeal
1 tablespoon baking powder
½ teaspoon salt
3 egg whites
2 tablespoons honey
3 tablespoons canola oil
1 cup skim milk

1. Mix dry ingredients (flour, cornmeal, baking powder, and salt) together.
2. In a separate bowl, blend the remaining ingredients and pour into the dry mixture. Blend thoroughly.
3. Pour batter into muffin tins that have been sprayed with vegetable oil spray or into cupcake papers.
4. Bake at 400° for 20 to 25 minutes or until brown.

Makes 1 dozen muffins, which can be served at breakfast, for snacks, or at other meals.

Nutritional information per serving: 117 calories; 17 grams carbohydrate; 3 grams protein; 4 grams total fat; trace saturated fat; trace cholesterol; 17 mg sodium; trace fiber.

TOFU ROLL-UPS

10 whole-wheat lasagna noodles, cooked according to package directions
1 lb soft tofu
2 egg whites
¼ cup, plus 3 tablespoons fat-free Parmesan cheese
1 cup fancy shredded fat-free mozzarella cheese
1 tablespoon dried basil
2 teaspoons ground oregano
1 teaspoon garlic salt
¼ teaspoon ground red pepper
¼ teaspoon black pepper
1 26¾ oz can of light spaghetti sauce

1. Blend tofu, egg whites, ¼ cup of Parmesan cheese, mozzarella cheese, and spices in a bowl until the mixture resembles a paste.

2. Spread lasagna noodles out on aluminum foil. Spread 3 tablespoons of the tofu mixture on a noodle, up to the edge. Repeat with other noodles. Roll up each noodle, and cut each roll in half.

3. Fill a large rectangular baking dish with spaghetti sauce. Place rolls in dish. Sprinkle with 3 tablespoons of Parmesan cheese.

4. Cover and bake in a 350° oven for 45 minutes.

Makes 6 servings.

Nutritional information per serving: 294 calories; 41 grams carbohydrate; 18 grams protein; 6 grams total fat; 4.5 grams saturated fat; 5 mg cholesterol; 943 mg sodium; 6 grams fiber.

LOW-FAT CREAMY ASPARAGUS SOUP

2 tablespoons olive oil
1 large onion, chopped

2 celery stalks, chopped
1 medium potato, peeled and grated
1 clove garlic, minced
2 teaspoons dried thyme
2 bay leaves
2 pounds fresh asparagus, sliced into ½ inch rounds,
with tips set aside
6 cups fat-free chicken broth
Salt and pepper to taste

1. In a large soup pot, sauté onions and celery in oil until onions are transparent and celery is tender.

2. Add remaining ingredients, except the asparagus tips. Cook over medium heat, covered, for 30 minutes.

3. Remove bay leaves. Puree mixture in a blender in batches until smooth. Return to the soup pot. Add salt and pepper to taste. Add the asparagus tips and simmer 4 minutes.

Makes 6 servings.

Nutritional information per serving: 122 calories; 15 grams carbohydrate; 7 grams protein; 5 grams total fat; trace saturated fat; 0 mg cholesterol; 403 mg sodium; 6 grams fiber.

THREE-BEAN SALAD

9-oz package of frozen green beans
¼ cup olive oil
¾ cup vinegar
Juice of ½ lemon
2 cloves garlic, minced
2 teaspoons sugar
1 15-oz can garbanzo beans, drained
1 15-oz can kidney beans, drained
1 medium onion, chopped
⅔ cup celery, chopped

1. Cook green beans according to package directions. Drain and let cool.

2. Combine remaining ingredients with green beans and mix well. Chill.

Makes 6 servings.

Nutritional information per serving: 262 calories; 33 grams carbohydrate; 11 grams protein; 3 grams total fat; 1 gram saturated fat; 0 mg cholesterol; 29 mg sodium; 6 grams fiber.

SHRIMP SCAMPI WITH BROCCOLI

1 tablespoon olive oil
1 tablespoon garlic, minced
½ teaspoon crushed red pepper
1 lb large shrimp, peeled and deveined
4 cups fresh broccoli florets
1 cup tomato sauce
¼ cup fresh basil, chopped
Salt and pepper to taste

1. Heat ½ tablespoon olive oil over medium heat in a skillet. Add garlic and red pepper. Cook one minute.

2. Add shrimp and season with salt. Sauté until shrimp turn pink, about 3 minutes. Transfer to a bowl and set aside.

3. Add the rest of the oil to the skillet with broccoli. Cook about 1 minute.

4. Add tomato sauce, cover and cook until broccoli is tender, about 3 minutes.

5. Add shrimp and basil and heat throughout. Season with salt and pepper if desired.

Makes 4 servings.

Nutritional information per serving: 169 calories; 13 grams carbohydrate; 20 grams protein; 5 grams total fat; trace saturated fat; 144 mg cholesterol; 145 mg sodium; 3 grams fiber.

NUT-CRUSTED FISH FILLETS

4 fish fillets (about 4 ounces each—perch, flounder, or catfish)
¼ cup toasted wheat germ
4 tablespoons crushed pecans or walnuts
1 garlic clove minced
¼ teaspoon salt
1 cup low-fat milk
Vegetable oil spray

1. In a shallow pan, combine wheat germ, crushed nuts, garlic, and salt.
2. Dip fillets in milk and dredge in wheat germ mixture.
3. Place fillets on a baking dish that has been sprayed with vegetable oil spray. Then spray each fillet with vegetable spray.
4. Bake at 425° for 15 minutes.

Makes 4 servings.

Nutritional information per serving: 202 calories; 8 grams carbohydrate; 26 grams protein; 7 grams total fat; trace saturated fat; 138 mg cholesterol; 123 mg sodium; 2 grams fiber.

TUNA NICOISE SALAD

3-oz can of tuna
½ cup cooked string beans (cold)
1 small boiled potato, sliced
Lettuce
Italian salad dressing

1. Arrange tuna, beans, and potato on a bed of lettuce.

2. Drizzle with 2 tablespoons salad dressing.

Makes 1 serving.

Nutritional information per serving: 248 calories; 28 grams carbohydrate; 25 grams protein; 3 grams total fat; trace saturated fat; 27 mg cholesterol; 574 mg sodium; 5 grams fiber.

REDUCED-FAT BLUE CHEESE DRESSING

1 cup fresh parsley
⅓ cup low-fat milk
½ cup fat-free yogurt
2 oz blue cheese, crumbled
1 tablespoon fresh squeezed lemon juice
1 tablespoon white balsamic vinegar
¼ teaspoon ground white pepper

1. Blend parsley on pulse setting until coarsely chopped.

2. Add remaining ingredients and blend until well mixed.

3. Store dressing in refrigerator for up to two weeks in an airtight container.

Makes 16 1-tablespoon servings

Nutritional information per serving: 24 calories; 1 gram carbohydrate; 1.5 grams protein; 1 gram total fat; trace saturated fat; 3 mg cholesterol; 11 mg sodium; 0 grams fiber.

LOW-FAT SLOPPY JOES

1 lb ground turkey
1 medium onion, chopped

1 teaspoon dry mustard
2 tablespoons brown sugar
1 tablespoon vinegar
1 12-oz bottle of chili sauce

1. Brown turkey in a non-stick skillet. Drain.
2. Add the remaining ingredients and simmer one hour. Serve on whole-wheat hamburger buns.

Makes 4 servings.

Nutritional information per serving: 264 calories; 30 grams carbohydrate; 19 grams protein; 8 grams total fat; 2 grams saturated fat; 0 mg cholesterol; 1171 mg sodium; 5 grams fiber.

BARBECUED CHICKEN BREASTS

1 small bottle reduced-fat Catalina salad dressing
2 tablespoons brown sugar
1 tablespoon teriyaki sauce
1 tablespoon light soy sauce
1 tablespoon barbecue sauce
4 skinless, boneless chicken breasts

1. Mix together salad dressing, brown sugar, teriyaki sauce, soy sauce, and barbecue sauce.
2. Place chicken in a shallow dish. Pour sauce mixture over chicken and let marinate in the refrigerator overnight or for several hours.
3. Grill chicken, basting occasionally with sauce.

Makes 4 servings.

Nutritional information per serving: 452 calories; 43 grams carbohydrate; 31 grams protein; 21 grams total fat; 4 grams saturated fat; 81 mg cholesterol; 696 mg sodium; 0 grams fiber.

ROSEMARY-SAUTÉED SPINACH

1 tablespoon sesame seed oil
2 tablespoons fresh rosemary, chopped
1 package (12 oz) prewashed fresh spinach leaves
4 tablespoons fat-free Parmesan cheese

1. Heat oil in a skillet over medium heat. Add rosemary and sauté until soft. Add spinach and sauté until wilted.
2. Serve and sprinkle Parmesan cheese over each serving.

Makes 4 servings.

Nutritional information per serving: 68 calories; 8 grams carbohydrate; 4 grams protein; 4 grams total fat; 1 gram saturated fat; 0mg cholesterol; 121 mg sodium; 1 gram fiber.

LOW-FAT FRIED BROWN RICE

2 cups cooked brown rice
½ cup frozen peas, thawed
2 tablespoons carrot, grated
¼ cup onion, chopped
1 tablespoon sesame seed oil
1 large egg, beaten
2 tablespoons light soy sauce
1 scallion, chopped

1. Combine rice, peas, carrot, and onion in a large mixing bowl.
2. Heat oil in a skillet. Add egg and cook until set. Chop egg into small pieces.
3. Add rice mixture to oil and egg. Stir in soy sauce. Heat throughout. Add scallions.

Makes 4 servings.

Nutritional information per serving: 182 calories; 26 grams carbohydrate; 4 grams protein; 6 grams total fat; 1 gram saturated fat; 53 mg cholesterol; 310 mg sodium; 3 grams fiber.

BAKED ALMOND FLAN

3 large eggs
1½ cups low-fat milk
1 cup evaporated fat-free milk
¼ cup sugar
¼ cup granulated Splenda
1 teaspoon almond extract
6 teaspoons slivered almonds

1. In a bowl, mix together eggs, low-fat milk, evaporated fat-free milk, sugar, Splenda, and extract. Blend well.

2. Divide mixture among 6 custard cups, filling each about ¾ full.

3. Top each with 1 teaspoon almonds.

4. Place custard dishes in a 9×13 baking dish and add hot water to reach one inch up the sides of the dishes.

5. Bake at 325° for about 1 hour or until a knife inserted in the center comes out clean. Remove custard dishes from water bath, and cool. Cover and chill in the refrigerator prior to serving.

Makes 6 servings.

Nutritional information per serving: 174 calories; 22 grams carbohydrate; 9 grams protein; 6 grams total fat; 1 gram saturated fat; 108 mg cholesterol; 132 mg sodium; 0 grams fiber.

QUICK SUGAR-FREE CHERRY COBBLER

1 can sugar-free cherry pie filling
6 sugar-free graham crackers, crushed
1 tablespoon trans-fat-free margarine

1. Put cherry pie filling in a glass baking dish.
2. Place cracker crumbs over the top.
3. Dot with margarine. Bake at 350° for 45 minutes.

Makes 4 servings.

Nutritional information per serving: 127 calories; 28 grams carbohydrate; 1 gram protein; 2 grams total fat; 0 grams saturated fat; 0 mg cholesterol; 55 mg sodium; 1 gram fiber.

CHAPTER 4

USING THE COUNTER

The *Foods that Combat Diabetes Counter* is the only compilation you'll find of diabetes-fighting foods. It contains data on calories, fat, saturated fat, trans fat, cholesterol, fiber, sugars, sodium, and the glycemic index for basic foods, brand-name foods, health foods, and fast foods—all right at your fingertips. Use this counter to make healthy choices, plan your meals, and ensure that you're getting the best nutrition from your food.

How to Find Your Foods

Foods are alphabetized in food categories as well as under individual categories so that you'll have no trouble finding whatever you want to look up. If you're looking for a particular food, look for it alphabetically under its category. Let's say, for example, you're looking for apples. Check the table of contents, where you'll find an alphabetized listing of food categories, and go to *fruits*. Turn to the page where the fruit listings begin and go to the *a*'s. Fruits are listed in alphabetical order, so it's easy to locate *apples*. Under *apples*, you'll find information for various types of apples, including raw, dehydrated, and applesauce. You'll be able to compare nutrient content of different preparations quickly and easily.

Fast foods are included, too—but only their healthier versions such as salads and sandwiches. Under fast foods, I've categorized them alphabetically for ease of use. You can look at each category and compare the nutrient quality of a Burger King selection to a McDonald's selection, for example. Generally, though, you're going to want to limit your intake of fast foods.

In the interest of good health, certain foods have been excluded from the counter, namely highly processed foods and those high in fat or sugar. Even though you'll find foods like cakes, ice cream, puddings, fast foods, and hot dogs in the counter, in most cases, only their low-fat and/or reduced sugar counterparts have been included.

Identifying Anti-Diabetes Nutrients

Each food entry lists the following information in this order: food name, serving size, caloric content, and the amount of each of the following (in grams, milligrams, micrograms, or other relevant measurement): protein, carbohydrate, fiber, sugars, total fat, saturated fat and trans fat, cholesterol, sodium, and the glycemic index (usually only if the food is a carbohydrate). Here's a closer look.

Serving Size

Serving size refers to a measurable amount of food as determined by the U.S. Department of Agriculture and the food industry.

Calories

This describes the amount of energy provided by one serving and can be used to help you accurately plan your meals if you're following a weight-reducing diet as part of your overall diabetes management or prevention plan.

Protein

Protein is important in managing diabetes because it helps control blood sugar when combined in a meal with carbohydrates. Most of the serving sizes for protein in this counter are given in 3- or 4-ounce servings. Protein should represent about 10 to 35 percent of your total daily calories. On a 1,500-calorie diet, for example, that translates to 150 to 525 calories a day, or 38 to 131 grams or 1.3 to 4.6 ounces of protein. If you eat according to the menu plan outlined in the previous chapter, you'll get adequate nutrition from this important food group.

Carbohydrate

Ideally, 45 to 65 percent of your total daily calories should come from carbohydrates, mainly natural, high-fiber sources of carbs. This equates to 675 to 975 calories, or 169 to 244 grams, on a 1,500-calorie diet. The grams of carbohydrate in the counter appear as total grams of carbohydrate. Although listed separately, fibers and sugars are counted as part of total carbohydrates.

Fiber

Hundreds of studies support the blood-sugar controlling power of fiber. In the counter, fiber content is presented in grams (g). Your best fiber bets will be found in cereals, grains, flours, fruits, nuts and seeds, vegetables, and some vegetarian-type fast foods. Look for foods that contain at least 2.5 to 3 grams of fiber per serving.

Sugars

There are two forms of sugar in the food we eat: *naturally occurring sugars* in fruits (fructose or fruit sugar), dairy products (lactose or milk sugar), and grains (maltose), and there are *added sugars* (white, brown, or powdered sugar as well as corn syrup solids) found in many processed foods. Added sugar is basically refined, simple sugar that has been introduced into the food during some stage of processing. Eating foods high in these sugars can lead not only to weight gain, but also to high blood sugar and insulin resistance.

Food labels lump natural sugars and added sugars together. In the counter, sugars in this case are counted in grams so that you can easily see the "total sugars" in your foods.

To distinguish between natural sugars and added sugars, you'll need to start by reading the ingredient list on the food label. Learn to differentiate between ingredients that are added sugars (corn syrup solids or sucrose) and natural sugars like lactose or fructose that are inherent in raw or basic foods. It may take some learning on your part to recognize sources of added versus natural sugars and may be a bit confusing at times because fructose is also used as an added sugar.

Please note that any product that contains natural sugars such as maltose, fructose, and lactose, and so on, may have no added sugar, but still contains natural sugars, and therefore has grams of sugar that can be counted.

Use the information in the "sugars" entry to avoid or limit simple sugars in your diet, and to ensure that you're getting healthy carbs in the right quantities. This information can also help you choose the most nutritious brands of your favorite food items (a breakfast cereal, for example, should contain between 0 and 5 grams of total sugars).

Recommended limits on sugar intake have not been

established. One health recommendation, however, is to cap your intake of added sugar at 10 percent or less than your total daily calories. For a 1,500 calorie diet, that would be 38 grams of sugar; for a 2,000 calorie diet, 50 grams.

Fat

The American Diabetes Association (ADA) recommends keeping your total fat intake between 25 and 35 percent of your daily calories. The goal is to limit the amount of saturated fats—that is, fat that is usually solid at room temperature—including most animal fats. In fact, the ADA recommends that saturated fat should be less than 7 percent of total calories for people with coronary heart disease, diabetes, or high LDL cholesterol. Much research strongly suggests that the right type of dietary fat (mainly unsaturated fats) plays a role in controlling diabetes. In the counter, fat content per serving is presented as total fat and saturated fat/trans fat. For example, for a serving of oatmeal, the entry is 3 grams (total fat) and 0/0 grams (saturated fat and trans fat). Use the counter to identify foods lowest in saturated fat and trans fat. Generally, you'll find them under fruits, vegetables, cereals, grains, soy foods, fish, poultry (white meat), and other low-fat entries.

Cholesterol

Cholesterol comes from two sources: the foods you eat and that which is formed in the body, primarily in the liver. Some cholesterol is beneficial, but too much in your blood could build up within the walls of your arteries, forming plaque and restricting blood flow. This condition can lead to heart disease, the number one killer of both men and women in the United States. People with diabetes are very prone to heart disease.

Making changes to your diet can help keep your

cholesterol levels under control by eating fewer high-cholesterol foods and watching your caloric intake. Cholesterol is found in eggs, meats, and high-fat dairy products. The American Diabetic Association recommends decreasing your cholesterol intake to less than 200 milligrams a day. Another smart move is to add plant stanols and sterols to your diet. These are found in the cholesterol-lowering spreads such as Benecol, Take Control, Smart Balance Plus, and in the dietary supplement Benecol SoftGels.

Sodium

In the diet, sodium is obtained mostly from salt and processed foods. Too much sodium in the body tends to narrow the diameter of blood vessels. When this happens, the heart has to work harder to pump the same amount of blood, and blood pressure goes up as a result. Excessive salt also makes the body retain too much water, and this may cause a rise in blood pressure.

Nearly 60 to 65 percent of people with diabetes have high blood pressure (hypertension), meaning a blood pressure reading that is higher than 140/90. However, medical experts don't know which comes first: diabetes or hypertension. Nor do they know exactly why diabetes keeps such close company with hypertension. But there are some theories. Factors that may give rise to high blood pressure in diabetes may include insulin resistance (in type 2 diabetes), obesity, excess secretion of stress hormones—and excess sodium in the diet.

The salt/blood pressure connection can be more dangerous in people with diabetes than in others without the disease. That's because many people with diabetes tend to be "sodium sensitive," which means they can get a rise in blood pressure at low daily salt intakes. Thus, cutting back on salt is usually a good idea.

The American Diabetes Association recommends limiting sodium intake to 2,400 mg (2.4 g) or sodium chloride (salt) to 6,000 mg (6 g) per day. The ADA gives two values here, because the element sodium makes up only about 40 percent of table salt. So all recommended daily allowances of sodium may be expressed as grams of table salt or as grams of sodium. (The counter gives grams of sodium.) One teaspoonful of table salt contains about 2 grams of sodium, and about 5 grams of salt.

If you have high blood pressure or kidney disease, a healthier target is less than 2,000 milligrams daily. The minimum requirement for adults is 500 milligrams a day, an amount provided by eating plain foods with no salt added.

One of the best ways to cut down on sodium intake is to avoid processed, snack, and fast foods, which contribute as much as 75 percent of the salt consumed in our diets. Other ways to reduce intake are to cook with only small amounts of salt and to season foods with sodium-free spices.

Glycemic Index (GI)

Not all carbohydrate foods are created equal; in fact, they act quite differently in the body. One way of describing this difference is through the glycemic index, or GI, of foods. As I mentioned earlier, the index ranks carbohydrates according to the rate at which they break down and release glucose into the bloodstream; the higher the GI, the greater the effect on glucose release and insulin secretion. Generally speaking, the more processed a food is, the higher its GI.

Foods on the index are rated numerically, with glucose at 100. The higher the number assigned to a food, the faster it converts to glucose. Foods with a rating of 70 or higher are generally considered high glycemic index foods; a rating of 50 to 69, moderate glycemic index foods; and below 50, low glycemic index foods. In the counter, only certain carbohydrate listings will contain a column for GI rankings, since foods containing little or no carbohydrate (such as meat, fish, eggs, avocado, wine, beer, spirits, and most vegetables) cannot have a GI value.

Abbreviations and Symbols
As you locate the foods in which you're interested, keep in mind the following abbreviations.

Measurements
fl oz	....	fluid ounce
g	....	gram
is	....	insignificant (in terms of a food's GI value)
mcg	....	microgram
mg	....	milligram
oz	....	ounce
tbsp	....	tablespoon
tsp	....	teaspoon
t	....	trace
w/	....	with
w/o	....	without

Food Descriptions and Nutrients
| 0 | .... | zero (no nutrient value) |
| na | .... | information not available *(Note: A designation of "na" does not mean an absence of a particular nutrient, only that analysis of that food for that nutrient is lacking.)* |

All the information in this counter is based on information from the United States government, from producers of brand-name foods, and from fast-food restaurant chains. Also consulted were numerous journal articles that analyzed the nutrient content of various foods.

This counter provides you with information to help you make the best possible food choices and take steps toward preventing and controlling diabetes. Take it wherever you go—to the grocery store, restaurants, and so forth—to make sure that you're eating right and eating well.

Food	Serving	Cal	Prot (g)	Carb (g)	Fiber (g)	Sugars (g)	Total Fat (g)	Sat/Trans Fat (g)	Chol (g)	Sod (mg)	GI
BEANS AND LENTILS											
Adzuki, boiled, w/salt	½ cup	147	9	28	8	na	t	t/0	0	281	35
Adzuki, boiled, w/o salt	½ cup	147	9	28	8	na	t	t/0	0	9	35
Beans, baked, canned, w/pork	½ cup	134	7	25	7	na	2	1/0	9	524	48
Beans, baked, canned, w/pork and tomato sauce	½ cup	124	7	25	6	na	1	t/0	9	557	48
Beans, baked, canned, w/pork and sweet sauce	½ cup	140	7	27	7	na	2	1/0	9	425	48
Beans, baked, canned, plain or vegetarian	½ cup	118	6	26	6	na	t	t/0	0	504	48
Black beans, boiled w/salt	½ cup	114	8	20	7.5	na	t	t/0	0	204	35
Black beans, boiled w/o salt	½ cup	114	8	20	7.5	na	t	t/0	0	1	35
Black beans, canned, Ranch Style (ConAgra)	½ cup	100	6	19	5	1	t	t/0	0	420	35
Broadbeans (fava), boiled, w/salt	½ cup	94	6	17	5	na	t	t/0	0	205	79
Broadbeans (fava), boiled, w/o salt	½ cup	94	6	17	5	na	t	t/0	0	4	79
Broadbeans (fava), canned	½ cup	91	7	16	5	na	t	t/0	0	580	79

76

Food	Serving	Cal	Prot (g)	Carb (g)	Fiber (g)	Sugars (g)	Total Fat (g)	Sat/Trans Fat (g)	Chol (g)	Sod (mg)	GI
Chickpeas (garbanzos), boiled, w/salt	½ cup	134	7	22	6	na	t	t/0	0	199	30
Chickpeas (garbanzos), boiled, w/o salt	½ cup	134	7	22	6	na	t	t/0	0	6	30
Chickpeas (garbanzos), canned	½ cup	143	6	27	5	na	t	t/0	0	359	35
Cranberry beans, boiled, w/salt	½ cup	120	8	22	9	na	t	t/0	0	210	35
Cranberry beans, boiled, w/o salt	½ cup	120	8	22	9	na	t	t/0	0	1	35
Cranberry beans, canned	½ cup	108	7	20	8	na	t	t/0	0	432	35
Great Northern beans, boiled, w/salt	½ cup	104	7	19	6	na	t	t/0	0	211	35
Great Northern beans, boiled, w/o salt	½ cup	104	7	19	6	na	t	t/0	0	2	35
Great Northern beans, canned	½ cup	149	10	28	6	na	t	t/0	0	5	35
Kidney beans, boiled, w/salt	½ cup	112	8	20	6	na	t	t/0	0	211	35
Kidney beans, boiled, w/o salt	½ cup	112	8	20	6	na	t	t/0	0	2	35

Food	Serving	Cal	Prot (g)	Carb (g)	Fiber (g)	Sugars (g)	Total Fat (g)	Sat/Trans Fat (g)	Chol (g)	Sod (mg)	GI
Kidney beans, canned	½ cup	104	7	19	4.5	na	t	t/0	0	444	40
Lentils, boiled, w/o salt	½ cup	115	9	20	8	na	t	t/0	0	2	29
Lentils, sprouted, raw	1 cup	82	7	17	na	na	t	t/0	0	8	29
Lima beans, baby, boiled, w/salt	½ cup	115	7	21	7	na	t	t/0	0	217	32
Lima beans, baby, boiled, w/o salt	½ cup	115	7	21	7	na	t	t/0	0	3	32
Lima beans, large, boiled, w/salt	½ cup	108	7	20	7	na	t	t/0	0	224	32
Lima beans, large, boiled, w/o salt	½ cup	108	7	20	7	na	t	t/0	0	2	32
Lima beans, large, canned	½ cup	95	6	18	6	na	t	t/0	0	405	32
Mung beans, boiled, w/salt	½ cup	106	7	19	8	na	t	t/0	0	240	31
Mung beans, boiled, w/o salt	½ cup	106	7	19	8	na	t	t/0	0	2	31
Navy beans, boiled, w/salt	½ cup	129	8	24	6	na	t	t/0	0	216	38
Navy beans, boiled, w/o salt	½ cup	129	8	24	6	na	t	t/0	0	1	38
Navy beans, canned	½ cup	148	10	27	7	na	t	t/0	0	587	38
Pink beans, boiled, w/salt	½ cup	126	8	24	4.5	na	t	t/0	0	201	na
Pink beans, boiled, w/o salt	½ cup	126	8	24	4.5	na	t	t/0	0	2	na

Food	Serving	Cal	Prot (g)	Carb (g)	Fiber (g)	Sugars (g)	Total Fat (g)	Sat/Trans Fat (g)	Chol (g)	Sod (mg)	GI
Pinto beans, boiled, w/salt	½ cup	117	7	22	7	na	t	t/0	0	203	39
Pinto beans, boiled, w/o salt	½ cup	117	7	22	7	na	t	t/0	0	2	39
Pinto beans, canned	½ cup	103	6	18	5.5	na	t	t/0	0	353	39
White beans (small), boiled, w/o salt	½ cup	127	8	23	9	na	t	t/0	0	2	35
White beans, boiled, w/salt	½ cup	124	9	23	6	na	t	t/0	0	217	35
White beans, boiled, w/o salt	½ cup	124	9	23	6	na	t	t/0	0	5	35
White beans, canned	½ cup	153	10	29	6	na	t	t/0	0	7	35

79

Food	Serving	Cal	Prot (g)	Carb (g)	Fiber (g)	Sugars (g)	Total Fat (g)	Sat/Trans Fat (g)	Chol (mg)	Sod (mg)
BEEF, LEAN CUTS										
Hamburger, 85% lean, pan-browned	3 oz	218	24	0	0	0	13	5/1	77	76
Hamburger, 90% lean, pan-browned	3 oz	196	24	0	0	0	10	4/t	76	74
Hamburger, 90% lean, broiled	3 oz	173	21	0	0	0	9	4/t	70	64
Hamburger, 95% lean, pan-browned	3 oz	164	25	0	0	0	6	3/t	76	72
Hamburger, 95% lean, broiled	3 oz	139	22	0	0	0	5	2/t	65	60
Bottom round, lean only, trimmed to 0" fat, all grades, roasted	4 oz	201	32	0	0	0	7	2.5/t	88	75
Bottom round, lean only, trimmed to 0" fat, choice, roasted	4 oz	210	31	0	0	0	9	3/t	117	41
Bottom round, lean only, trimmed to 0" fat, select, roasted	4 oz	194	33	0	0	0	6	2/t	88	75
Bottom round, lean only, trimmed to ¼" fat, all grades, roasted	4 oz	214	33	0	0	0	8	3/t	88	75

Food	Serving	Cal	Prot (g)	Carb (g)	Fiber (g)	Sugars (g)	Total Fat (g)	Sat/Trans Fat (g)	Chol (mg)	Sod (mg)
Bottom round, lean only, trimmed to ¼" fat, choice, roasted	4 oz	224	33	0	0	0	9	3/t	88	75
Bottom round, lean only, trimmed to ¼" fat, select, roasted	4 oz	203	33	0	0	0	7	2/t	88	75
Bottom round, lean and fat, trimmed to ⅛" fat, all grades, roasted	4 oz	247	31	0	0	0	13	5/t	85	40
Bottom round, lean and fat, trimmed to ⅛" fat, select, roasted	4 oz	240	31	0	0	0	12	5/t	90	40
Eye of the round, lean only, trimmed to 0" fat, all grades, roasted	4 oz	184	33	0	0	0	5	2/t	62	43
Eye of the round, lean only, trimmed to 0" fat, choice, roasted	4 oz	184	33	0	0	0	6	2/t	78	43
Eye of the round, lean only, trimmed to 0" fat, select, roasted	4 oz	176	33	0	0	0	4	1/t	78	66
Eye of the round, lean and fat, trimmed to 0" fat, select, roasted	4 oz	182	33	0	0	0	5	2/t	78	70

Food	Serving	Cal	Prot (g)	Carb (g)	Fiber (g)	Sugars (g)	Total Fat (g)	Sat/Trans Fat (g)	Chol (mg)	Sod (mg)
Flank steak, lean only, trimmed to 0" fat, choice, broiled	4 oz	235	31	0	0	0	11.5	5/t	76	94
Flank steak, lean and fat, trimmed to 0" fat, choice, broiled	4 oz	256	30	0	0	0	14	6/t	77	92
Porterhouse steak, lean only, trimmed to 0" fat, all grades, broiled	4 oz	240	30	0	0	0	13	4/t	70	78
Porterhouse steak, lean only, trimmed to 0" fat, choice, broiled	4 oz	254	29	0	0	0	14.5	5/t	74	78
Porterhouse steak, lean only, trimmed to 0" fat, select, broiled	4 oz	220	30	0	0	0	10	4/t	66	78
Porterhouse steak, lean only, trimmed to ¼" fat, choice, broiled	4 oz	244	30	0	0	0	13	4/t	78	78
Porterhouse steak, lean only, trimmed to ¼" fat, select, broiled	4 oz	230	31	0	0	0	11	4/t	66	78
Round, tip round, lean only, trimmed to 0" fat, all grades, roasted	4 oz	199	33	0	0	0	7	2/t	92	74

Food	Serving	Cal	Prot (g)	Carb (g)	Fiber (g)	Sugars (g)	Total Fat (g)	Sat/Trans Fat (g)	Chol (mg)	Sod (mg)
Round, tip round, lean only, trimmed to 0" fat, choice, roasted	4 oz	204	33	0	0	0	7	2.5/t	92	74
Round, tip round, lean only, trimmed to 0" fat, select, roasted	4 oz	193	32.5	0	0	0	6	2/t	92	74
Round, tip round, lean only, trimmed to ¼" fat, all grades, roasted	4 oz	210	32.5	0	0	0	8	3/t	92	74
Round, tip round, lean only, trimmed to ¼" fat, choice, roasted	4 oz	213	32.5	0	0	0	8	3/t	92	74
Round, tip round, lean only, trimmed to ¼" fat, select, roasted	4 oz	204	32.5	0	0	0	7	2.5/t	92	74
Round, tip round, lean and fat, trimmed to 0" fat, all grades, roasted	4 oz	216	32	0	0	0	9	3/t	92	73
Round, tip round, lean and fat, trimmed to 0" fat, choice, roasted	4 oz	227	32	0	0	0	10	4/t	93	73

Food	Serving	Cal	Prot (g)	Carb (g)	Fiber (g)	Sugars (g)	Total Fat (g)	Sat/Trans Fat (g)	Chol (mg)	Sod (mg)
Round, tip round, lean and fat, trimmed to 0" fat, select, roasted	4 oz	211	32	0	0	0	8	3/t	92	73
Round, tip round, lean and fat, trimmed to ⅛" fat, all grades, roasted	4 oz	248	31	0	0	0	13	5/t	93	71
Round, tip round, lean and fat, trimmed to ⅛" fat, all grades, roasted	4 oz	258	31	0	0	0	14	5/t	93	71
Round, tip round, lean and fat, trimmed to ⅛" fat, all grades, roasted	4 oz	238	31	0	0	0	12	4/t	93	73
T-bone steak, lean only, trimmed to 0" fat, all grades, broiled	4 oz	214	29	0	0	0	10	3.5/t	62	80
T-bone steak, lean only, trimmed to 0" fat, choice, broiled	4 oz	224	29	0	0	0	11	4/t	63	80
T-bone steak, lean only, trimmed to 0" fat, select, broiled	4 oz	201	29	0	0	0	8	3/t	61	80
T-bone steak, lean only, trimmed to ¼" fat, all grades, broiled	4 oz	229	31	0	0	0	11	4/t	65	85

84

Food	Serving	Cal	Prot (g)	Carb (g)	Fiber (g)	Sugars (g)	Total Fat (g)	Sat/Trans Fat (g)	Chol (mg)	Sod (mg)
T-bone steak, lean only, trimmed to ¼" fat, choice, broiled	4 oz	232	30	0	0	0	11	4/t	67	87
T-bone steak, lean only, trimmed to ¼" fat, select, broiled	4 oz	224	31	0	0	0	10	4/t	60	80
Tenderloin, lean only, trimmed to 0" fat, choice, broiled (filet mignon, beef medallions)	4 oz	240	32	0	0	0	11	4/t	95	71
Top round, lean only, trimmed to 0" fat, all grades, braised (London broil)	4 oz	226	41	0	0	0	6	2/t	102	51
Top round, lean and fat, trimmed to 0" fat, choice, braised (London broil)	4 oz	245	40	0	0	0	8	3/t	102	51
Top round, lean only, trimmed to 0" fat, select, braised (London broil)	4 oz	215	41	0	0	0	5	1.5/t	102	51
Top round, lean and fat, trimmed to 0" fat, select, braised (London broil)	4 oz	227	41	0	0	0	6	2/t	102	51

Food	Serving	Cal	Prot (g)	Carb (g)	Fiber (g)	Sugars (g)	Total Fat (g)	Sat/Trans Fat (g)	Chol (mg)	Sod (mg)
Top round, lean only, trimmed to ¼" fat, all grades, braised (London broil)	4 oz	231	41	0	0	0	6	2/t	102	51
Top round, lean only, trimmed to ¼" fat, all grades, broiled (London broil)	4 oz	204	36	0	0	0	5.5	2/t	95	69
Top round, lean and fat only, trimmed to ⅛" fat, select, broiled (London broil)	4 oz	222	35	0	0	0	8	3/t	96	68
Top sirloin, lean only, trimmed to 0" fat, all grades, broiled	4 oz	216	34	0	0	0	8	3/t	101	75
Top sirloin, lean only, trimmed to 0" fat, choice, broiled	4 oz	227	34	0	0	0	9	3.5/t	101	75
Top sirloin, lean only, trimmed to 0" fat, select, broiled	4 oz	204	34	0	0	0	6	2.5/t	101	75
Top sirloin, lean only, trimmed to ¼" fat, all grades, broiled	4 oz	221	34	0	0	0	8	3/t	101	75
Top sirloin, lean only, trimmed to ¼" fat, choice, broiled	4 oz	229	34	0	0	0	9	3.5/t	101	75

Food	Serving	Cal	Prot (g)	Carb (g)	Fiber (g)	Sugars (g)	Total Fat (g)	Sat/Trans Fat (g)	Chol (mg)	Sod (mg)
Top sirloin, lean only, trimmed to ¼" fat, select, broiled	4 oz	211	34	0	0	0	7	3/t	101	75
Top sirloin, lean and fat, trimmed to 0" fat, all grades, broiled	4 oz	244	33	0	0	0	11	4.5/t	101	74
Top sirloin, lean and fat, trimmed to 0" fat, choice, broiled	4 oz	260	33	0	0	0	13	5/t	101	73
Top sirloin, lean and fat, trimmed to 0" fat, select, broiled	4 oz	221	34	0	0	0	8.5	3/t	101	74

Food	Serving	Cal	Prot (g)	Carb (g)	Fiber (g)	Sugars (g)	Total Fat (g)	Sat/Trans Fat (g)	Chol (g)	Sod (mg)	GI
BEVERAGES/ALCOHOLIC/BEER											
Beer, light	1 can or bottle, 12 fl oz	99	1	5	0	t	0	0/0	0	14	110
Beer, nonalcoholic (O'Doul's)	1 can or bottle, 12 fl oz	65	1	13	0	na	0	0/0	0	na	na
Beer, low carb	1 can or bottle, 12 fl oz	96	t	2.5	0	t	0	0/0	0	na	na
Beer, regular	1 can or bottle, 12 fl oz	146	1	13	0	t	0	0/0	0	18	110
BEVERAGES/ALCOHOLIC/ DISTILLED LIQUORS											
80 proof	1 jigger, 1.5 fl oz	97	0	t	0	na	0	0/0	0	0	0

Food	Serving	Cal	Prot (g)	Carb (g)	Fiber (g)	Sugars (g)	Total Fat (g)	Sat/Trans Fat (g)	Chol (g)	Sod (mg)	GI
90 proof	1 jigger, 1.5 fl oz	110	0	t	0	na	0	0/0	0	0	0
100 proof	1 jigger, 1.5 fl oz	124	0	t	0	na	0	0/0	0	0	0
BEVERAGES/ALCOHOLIC/WINE											
Champagne	1 wine glass, 3.5 fl oz	72	0		0		0	0/0	0	na	0
Dessert, dry	1 wine glass, 3.5 fl oz	130	t	4	0	na	0	0/0	0	9	0
Dessert, sweet	1 wine glass, 3.5 fl oz	158	t	12	0	na	0	0/0	0	9	0
Nonalcoholic	1 wine glass, 3.5 fl oz	6	t	1	0	0	0	0/0	0	2	na

Food	Serving	Cal	Prot (g)	Carb (g)	Fiber (g)	Sugars (g)	Total Fat (g)	Sat/Trans Fat (g)	Chol (g)	Sod (mg)	GI
Red	1 wine glass, 3.5 fl oz	74	t	2	0	na	0	0/0	0	5	0
Rose	1 wine glass, 3.5 fl. oz.	73	t	1	0	na	0	0/0	0	5	0
Sherry (medium)	1 wine glass, 3.5 fl oz	58	0	2.5	0	na	0	0/0	0	5	0
White	1 wine glass, 3.5 fl oz	70	t	1	0	na	0	0/0	0	5	0
Wine cooler	1 drink, 7 fl oz	520	1	80	0	na	0	0/0	0	na	na
BEVERAGES/COFFEE											
Brewed	1 cup	5	t	t	0	0	0	0/0	0	5	0
Brewed, decaf	1 cup	5	t	t	0	0	0	0/0	0	5	0

Food	Serving	Cal	Prot (g)	Carb (g)	Fiber (g)	Sugars (g)	Total Fat (g)	Sat/Trans Fat (g)	Chol (g)	Sod (mg)	GI
Chicory added, instant	1 cup	10	t	2	0	0	0	0/0	0	14	0
Espresso, restaurant prepared	100 grams	9	t	1.5	0	0	0	0/0	0	14	0
French vanilla flavor, sugar-free, fat-free, instant, prepared	1 cup	25	t	5	t	t	0	0/0	0	65	0
French mocha flavor, sugar-free, fat-free, instant, prepared	1 cup	24	t	5	1	t	0	0/0	0	36	0
Instant	1 cup	5	t	t	0	0	0	0/0	0	7	0
Instant, decaf	1 cup	4	T	T	0	0	0	0/0	0	0	0
BEVERAGES/NON-CALORIC											
Carbonated/mineral water	1 cup	0	0	0	0	0	0	0/0	0	2	0
Club soda	1 can (12 fl oz)	0	0	0	0	0	0	0/0	0	75	0
Diet soft drinks	1 can (12 fl oz)	4	t	t	0	t	0	0/0	0	35	0

Food	Serving	Cal	Prot (g)	Carb (g)	Fiber (g)	Sugars (g)	Total Fat (g)	Sat/Trans Fat (g)	Chol (g)	Sod (mg)	GI
Energy drink, Red Bull, sugar free	1 can (8.3 fl oz)	13	.6	1.75	0	0	t	0/0	0	210	0
Lemonade, low-calorie, w/ aspartame, prepared	1 cup	5	0	1	0	0	0	0/0	0	5	0
Municipal water	1 cup	0	0	0	0	0	0	0	0	5	0
Soft drink mix, tropical flavor, unsweetened, powder	1 serving	1	0	t	0	t		0/0	0	15	0
BEVERAGES/TEA											
Brewed	1 cup	2	0	t	0	0	0	0/0	0	7	0
Brewed, decaf	1 cup	2	0	1	0	0	0	0/0	0	7	0
Chamomile, brewed	1 cup	2	0	t	0	0	0	0/0	0	2	0
Herbal, brewed	1 cup	2	0	t	0	0	0	0/0	0	2	0
Instant, unsweetened	1 cup	2	0	t	0	0	0	0/0	0	7	0
Instant, unsweetened, lemon-flavored	1 cup	5	0	1	0	0	0	0/0	0	14	0

Food	Serving	Cal	Prot (g)	Carb (g)	Fiber (g)	Sugars (g)	Total Fat (g)	Sat/Trans Fat (g)	Chol (g)	Sod (mg)	GI
Sugar-free, low-calorie, w/ aspartame	1 cup	3	t	t	0	t	0	0/0	0	2	0
Sugar-free, low-calorie, lemon-flavored w/saccharin	1 cup	5	0	1	0	0	0	0/0	0	24	0
BREADS, BAGELS, MUFFINS, AND ROLLS											
Breads and Bagels											
Bagel, oat bran, 3"	3" dia.	145	6	31	2	1	1	t/t	0	289	72
Bagel, plain, enriched, 3"	3" dia.	190	7	37	2	na	2	t/t	0	368	72
Cracked wheat bread	1 slice	65	2	12	1.4	1	1	t/t	0	135	58
Egg bread	1 slice	113	4	19	1	1	2	1/na	20	197	na
Mixed grain bread	1 slice	65	3	12	2	3	1	t/na	0	127	65
Oat bran bread	1 slice	71	3	12	1	2	1	t/na	0	122	47
Oat bran bread, reduced-calorie	1 slice	46	2	10	3	1	1	t/na	0	81	47
Oatmeal bread	1 slice	73	2	13	1	2	1	t/na	0	162	65
Oatmeal bread, reduced-calorie	1 slice	48	2	10	na	na	t	t/na	0	89	65

Food	Serving	Cal	Prot (g)	Carb (g)	Fiber (g)	Sugars (g)	Total Fat (g)	Sat/Trans Fat (g)	Chol (g)	Sod (mg)	GI
Pita bread, whole wheat	4" dia.	74	3	15	2	na	1	t/na	0	149	57
Protein bread	1 slice	47	2	8	1	t	t	t/na	0	104	na
Pumpernickel bread	1 slice	65	2	12	2	t	t	t/na	0	174	50
Raisin bread	1 slice	71	2	14	1	1	1	t/na	0	101	63
Rice bran bread	1 slice	66	2	12	1	1	1	t/na	0	119	61
Rye bread	1 slice	83	3	15	2	1	t	t/na	0	211	50
Rye bread, reduced calorie	1 slice	47	2	9	3	.5	t	t/na	0	93	50
Tortilla, corn (not fried)	1 medium (6" dia.)	42	1	9	1	na	.5	t/na	na	31	52
Tortilla, whole-wheat	1 medium (7" dia.)	84	3	23	2	na	.5	t/na	na	196	30
Wheatberry bread	1 slice	65	2	12	1	na	1	t/na	0	132	58
Wheat bran bread	1 slice	89	3	17	1.4	3.5	1	t/na	0	175	58
Wheat bread, reduced-calorie	1 slice	46	2	10	3	3	t	t/na	0	118	na

Food	Serving	Cal	Prot (g)	Carb (g)	Fiber (g)	Sugars (g)	Total Fat (g)	Sat/Trans Fat (g)	Chol (g)	Sod (mg)	GI
Wheat germ bread	1 slice	73	3	13.5	t	4	t	t/na	0	155	58
Whole-wheat bread	1 slice	69	3	13	2	1.5	1	t/na	0	148	58
Bread, white	1 slice	67	2	12	t	1	1	t/na	0	134	73
Muffins											
English muffin, wheat	1 muffin	127	5	26	3	1	1	t/na	0	218	77
English muffin, whole-wheat	1 muffin	134	6	27	4	5	1	t/na	0	420	77
Mixed grain, includes granola	1 muffin	155	6	31	2	na	1	t/na	0	275	60
Oat bran muffin	1 small	178	5	32	3	.5	5	1.na	0	259	60
Oat bran muffin	1 mini	46	1	8	1	5	1	t/na	0	67	
Oat bran, prepared from recipe, made w/low-fat milk (2%)	1 muffin	169	4	24	2	na	7	1/na	22	266	60
Wheat bran, toaster-type w/raisins	1 muffin	106	2	19	3	5	3	t/na	6	178	na
Rolls											
Biscuits, buttermilk, refrigerated dough, lower fat, baked	1 biscuit (2½" dia.)	63	2	1,225	t	2	1	t/na	na	305	70

95

Food	Serving	Cal	Prot (g)	Carb (g)	Fiber (g)	Sugars (g)	Total Fat (g)	Sat/Trans Fat (g)	Chol (g)	Sod (mg)	GI
Biscuits, plain, refrigerated dough, higher fat, baked	1 biscuit (2½" dia.)	95	2	13	t	2	4	1/1	0	292	70
Biscuits, plain or buttermilk, prepared from recipe	1 biscuit (4" dia.)	357	7	45	1	2	17	4/na	3	586	70
Biscuits, plain or buttermilk, commercially prepared	1 biscuit, large	281	5	37	1	3	13	2/na	0	810	70
Cornbread, prepared from dry mix	1 piece	188	4	29	1	na	6	2/na	37	467	72
Cornbread, prepared from recipe, made w/low-fat (2%) milk	1 piece	173	4	28	na	na	5	1/na	26	428	72
Dinner rolls (includes brown-and-serve)	1 roll (1 oz)	84	2	14	1	1.5	2	t/na	1	146	na
Dinner rolls, whole wheat	1 roll, medium (2½" dia.)	96	3	18	3	3	2	t/na	0	172	na
French baguette	1 slice	185	8	36	2	2	1	t/na	0	416	70

Food	Serving	Cal	Prot (g)	Carb (g)	Fiber (g)	Sugars (g)	Total Fat (g)	Sat/Trans Fat (g)	Chol (g)	Sod (mg)	GI
French rolls	1 roll	105	3	19	1	t	2	t/na	0	231	na
French toast, frozen, ready-to-heat	1 piece	126	4	19	1	na	4	1/na	48	292	na
Hamburger or hot dog bun, mixed-grain	1 bun	113	4	19	2	3	3	1/na	0	197	61
Hamburger or hot dog bun, plain	1 bun	120	4	21	1	3	2	.5/na	0	206	61
Hamburger or hot dog bun, reduced-calorie	1 bun	84	4	18	3	2	1	t/na	0	190	na
Italian bread	1 slice, large (4½" × 3¾" × ¾")	81	3	15	1	t	1	t/na	0	175	na
Italian bread, garlic, crusty (Pepperidge Farm)	1 serving	186	4	21	na	na	10	2/na	6	200	na
Kaiser rolls	1 roll (3½" dia.)	167	6	30	1	1	2.5	t/na	0	310	73

Food	Serving	Cal	Prot (g)	Carb (g)	Fiber (g)	Sugars (g)	Total Fat (g)	Sat/Trans Fat (g)	Chol (g)	Sod (mg)	GI
Rye dinner roll	1 roll, large (3½" to 4" dia.)	123	4	23	2	.5	1.5	t/na	0	384	na
Stuffing, bread	½ cup	177	3	22	3	2	9	2/na	0	543	74
Stuffing, chicken flavor	½ cup	107	4	20	1	3	1	na/na	1	429	74
Stuffing, cornbread	½ cup	179	3	22	3	4	9	2/na	0	455	74
Taco shells, baked	1 medium (5" dia.)	59	1	8	1	t	3	.5/.6	0	49	68
CEREALS, COLD											
100% Bran Cereal (Post)	⅓ cup	82	4	22	8	7	t	t/na	0	120	na
All-Bran (Kellogg's)	½ cup	81	4	23	10	6	1	t/0	0	80	42
All-Bran with Extra Fiber (Kellogg's)	½ cup	50	3	20	13	t	1	t/0	0	124	42
All-Bran Bran Buds (Kellogg's)	⅓ cup	74	2	24	13	8	t	t/0	0	201	58
Banana Nut Crunch (Post)	1 cup	249	5	44	4	12	6	t/na	0	253	na
Basic 4 (General Mills)	1 cup	202	4	42	3	14	3	t/0	0	316	na

98

Food	Serving	Cal	Prot (g)	Carb (g)	Fiber (g)	Sugars (g)	Total Fat (g)	Sat/Trans Fat (g)	Chol (g)	Sod (mg)	GI
Bran Flakes (Post)	¾ cup	96	3	24	5	6	1	0/0	0	220	74
Cheerios, multi-grain (General Mills)	1 cup	108	2	24	3	6	1	t/0	0	201	74
Complete Oat Bran Flakes (Kellogg's)	¾ cup	105	3	23	4	6	1	t/0	0	210	74
Complete Wheat Bran Flakes (Kellogg's)	¾ cup	92	3	23	5	5	t	t/0	0	207	74
Cracklin' Oat Bran (Kellogg's)	¾ cup	225	5	39	6	17	8	2/t	0	157	na
Crunchy Bran (Quaker)	¾ cup	90	1	23	5	6	1	0/0	0	232	na
Fiber One (General Mills)	½ cup	59	2	24	14	0	t	t/0	0	129	na
Fruit & Fibre (Post)	1 cup	212	4	42	5	16	3	t/na	0	280	na
Granola w/raisins, low-fat (Kellogg's)	⅔ cup	231	5	48	3	17	3	1/t	0	148	na
Granola w/o raisins, low-fat (Kellogg's)	½ cup	209	5	44	3	3	3	1/t	0	135	na
Granola w/raisins, low-fat (Quaker)	½ cup	195	4	41	17	3	3	t/na	1	119	na

Food	Serving	Cal	Prot (g)	Carb (g)	Fiber (g)	Sugars (g)	Total Fat (g)	Sat/Trans Fat (g)	Chol (g)	Sod (mg)	GI
Grape Nuts (Post)	½ cup	208	6	47	5	7	1	t/na	0	354	71
Grape Nuts Flakes (Post)	¾ cup	106	3	24	3	5	t	t/na	0	140	>70
Great Grains (Post)	⅔ cup	204	4	40	4	13	5	t/na	0	156	na
Healthy Choice Almond Crunch w/Raisins (Kellogg's)	1 cup	198	5	43	5	15	3	t/na	0	215	na
Kashi GoLean (Kellogg's)	1 cup	148	14	30	10	6	15	t/0	0	86	<55
Kashi GoLean Crunch (Kellogg's)	1 cup	200	9	36	8	13	3	t/0	0	204	<55
Kashi Good Friends (Kellogg's)	1 cup	167	5	43	12	9	2	t/0	0	129	<55
Kashi Heart to Heart (Kellogg's)	1 cup	115	4	25	5	7	2	t/0	0	1	<55
Kashi Seven in the Morning (Kellogg's)	½ cup	178	6	41	6	2.5	1	t/0	0	224	na
Life (Quaker)	¾ cup	120	3	25	2	6	1	t/na	0	164	56–69
Multi-Bran Chex (General Mills)	1 cup	180	4	46	7	11	1	t/0	0	342	56–69
Mueslix (Kellogg's)	⅔ cup	197	5	40	4	17	3	t/0	0	171	<55

Food	Serving	Cal	Prot (g)	Carb (g)	Fiber (g)	Sugars (g)	Total Fat (g)	Sat/Trans Fat (g)	Chol (g)	Sod (mg)	GI
Product 19 (Kellogg's)	1 cup	100	2	25	1	4	t	t/0	0	207	na
Raisin Bran (Kellogg's)	1 cup	195	5	47	7	20	2	t/0	0	362	61
Raisin Bran (Post)	1 cup	187	5	46	8	20	1	t/na	0	360	61
Raisin Nut Bran (General Mills)	¾ cup	209	4	42	5	15	4	.5/.5	0	250	na
Rice Chex (General Mills)	1¼ cup	120	2	27	t	2	.5	t/0	0	292	89
Shredded Wheat (Post)	2 biscuits	155	5	36	6	t	1	t/0	0	3	75
Shredded wheat, spoon sized (Post)	1 cup	167	5	41	6	t	t	t/na	0	3	75
Shredded Wheat 'N Bran (Post)	1¼ cup	197	7	47	8	t	1	t/na	0	3	75
Smart Start (Kellogg's)	1 cup	182	3	43	2	16	t	t/0	0	281	na
Smart Start w/soy protein (Kellogg's)	1 cup	202	10	40	4	14	1.5	t/0	0	261	na
Smart Start Healthy Heart (Kellogg's)	1¼ cup	225	7	46	6	17	3	.5/t	0	139	na
Special K (Kellogg's)	1 cup	117	7	22	t	4	t	t/0	0	224	69

101

Food	Serving	Cal	Prot (g)	Carb (g)	Fiber (g)	Sugars (g)	Total Fat (g)	Sat/Trans Fat (g)	Chol (g)	Sod (mg)	GI
Special K Low Carb Lifestyle (Kellogg's)	¾ cup	101	10	14	5	2	3	.5/0	0	110	na
Total, Corn Flakes (General Mills)	1⅓ cup	112	2	26	t	3	t	t/0	0	209	76
Total, Raisin Bran (General Mills)	1 cup	171	4	41	5	20	1	t/0	0	239	61
Total, whole grain (General Mills)	¾ cup	97	2	22	2	5	t	t/0	0	192	70
Uncle Sam	1 cup	237	9	36	11	1	6	t/na	0	113	na
Wheaties (General Mills)	1 cup	110	3	24	3	4	1	t/0	0	210	na
CEREALS, HOT											
Corn grits, white, w/o salt	½ cup	73	2	16	t	t	t	t/0	0	0	68
Corn grits, yellow, w/o salt	½ cup	73	2	16	t	t	t	t/0	0	0	68
Corn grits, instant, butter flavor (Quaker)	1 packet	101	2	21	1	t	1	t/0	0	323	68
Corn grits, instant, cheddar cheese flavor (Quaker)	1 packet	99	2	20	1	t	2	t/na	0	510	na
Corn grits, instant, plain (Quaker)	1 packet	89	2	21	1	t	t	t/0	0	289	68
Cream of rice, w/o salt	½ cup	63	1	14	t	t	t	t/0	0	1	na

Food	Serving	Cal	Prot (g)	Carb (g)	Fiber (g)	Sugars (g)	Total Fat (g)	Sat/Trans Fat (g)	Chol (g)	Sod (mg)	GI
Cream of wheat, instant, w/o salt	½ cup	77	2	16	1	t	t	t/0	0	4	66
Cream of wheat, mix 'n eat, plain	1 packet	102	3	21	t	t	t	t/0	0	241	66
Cream of wheat, quick, w/o salt	½ cup	64	2	13	1	t	t	t/0	0	69	66
Cream of wheat, regular, w/o salt	½ cup	66	2	14	1	t	t	t/0	0	1	66
Farina, w/o salt	½ cup	58	2	12	2	t	t	t/0	0	0	na
Malt-O-Meal, plain, w/o salt	½ cup	61	2	13	.5	t	t	t/0	0	1	na
Maypo, w/o salt	¾ cup	128	4	24	4	11	2	0/0	0	7	na
Multi-grain oatmeal, dry	½ cup	133	5	29	2.5	0	1	0/0	0	1	na
Nestum	½ cup	95	3	17	3.5	0	t	0/0	0	5	na
Oats, instant, plain	½ cup	69	3	12	2	0	1	t/0	0	188	65
Oats, instant, w/bran and raisins	1 packet	158	5	30	6	0	2	t/0	0	248	na
Oats, old-fashioned, w/o salt	½ cup	150	5	27	4	0	3	0/0	0	0	75
Oat bran	½ cup	146	7	25	6	0	3	t/0	0	2	50
Oatmeal, instant, w/apples and cinnamon	1 packet	125	3	26	2.5	12	1	t/0	0	121	na

Food	Serving	Cal	Prot (g)	Carb (g)	Fiber (g)	Sugars (g)	Total Fat (g)	Sat/Trans Fat (g)	Chol (g)	Sod (mg)	GI
Oatmeal, instant, w/cinnamon and spice, prepared w/water	1 packet	177	5	35	3	16	2	t/0	0	280	na
Oatmeal, microwave, brown sugar and cinnamon	1 packet	155	4	31	3	12	2	t/0	0	255	na
Oatmeal, instant, w/maple and brown sugar, prepared w/water	1 packet	153	4	31	3	na	2	t/0	0	234	na
Oatmeal, microwave, brown sugar and cinnamon	1 packet	155	4	31	3	12	2	t/0	0	255	na
Oatmeal, microwave, cinnamon and double raisin	1 packet	169	4	35	3	15	2	t/0	0	275	na
Ralston, w/o salt	½ cup	67	3	14	3	na	t	t/0	0	3	na
Roman Meal, plain, cooked, w/salt	½ cup	74	3	16.5	4	na	t	t/0	0	99	na
Roman Meal, plain, cooked, w/o salt	½ cup	74	3	16.5	4	na	t	t/0	0	1	na
Roman Meal with Oats, w/salt	½ cup	85	4	17	4	na	1	t/0	0	270	na
Roman Meal with Oats, w/salt	½ cup	85	4	17	3.5	na	1	t/0	0	5	na
Wheatena	½ cup	68	2	14	3	t	t	t/0	0	289	na

Food	Serving	Cal	Prot (g)	Carb (g)	Fiber (g)	Sugars (g)	Total Fat (g)	Sat/Trans Fat (g)	Chol (g)	Sod (mg)	GI
Whole-wheat, hot natural cereal, w/salt	½ cup	75	2.5	17	2	t	t	t/0	0	282	<55
Whole-wheat, hot natural cereal, w/o salt	½ cup	75	2.5	17	2	t	t	t/0	0	0	<55
CEREAL BARS											
Cereal bar, fruit	1 bar (1 oz)	103	1	20	1	na	2	t/0	0	83	<55
Cereal bar, mixed berry	1 bar (1 oz)	104	1	20	.5	9	2	t/0	0	83	<55
Chocolate chip crisped rice bar	1 bar (1 oz)	113	1	20	1	na	3	1/0	0	78	na
Granola bar, hard, almond	1 bar	119	2	15	1	na	6	3/na	0	61	87
Granola bar, hard, chocolate chip	1 bar	105	2	17	1	na	4	3/na	0	83	87
Granola bar, hard, peanut	1 bar (1 oz)	136	3	18	1	10	6	1/na	0	79	87
Granola bar, hard, peanut butter	1 bar (0.85 oz)	116	2	15	1	na	6	1/na	0	68	87

Food	Serving	Cal	Prot (g)	Carb (g)	Fiber (g)	Sugars (g)	Total Fat (g)	Sat/Trans Fat (g)	Chol (g)	Sod (mg)	GI
Granola bar, hard, plain	1 bar (1 oz)	132	3	18	1	na	6	1/na	0	82	87
Granola bar, soft, chocolate chip w/milk chocolate coating	1 bar (1.25 oz)	163	2	22	1	na	9	5/na	2	70	87
Granola bar, soft, chocolate chip w/milk chocolate coating	1 bar (1 oz)	130	2	18	1	na	7	4/na	1	56	87
Granola bar, soft, peanut butter w/milk chocolate coating	1 bar (1.3 oz)	188	4	20	1	na	12	6/na	4	71	87
Granola bar, soft, chocolate chip, uncoated	1 bar (1.5 oz)	181	3	30	2	12	7	4/na	0	117	87
Granola bar, soft, chocolate chip, uncoated	1 bar (1 oz)	118	2	19	1	8	5	3/na	0	76	87
Granola bar, soft, chocolate chip, graham and marshmallow, uncoated	1 bar (1 oz)	120	2	20	1	na	4	3/na	0	88	87
Granola bar, soft, nut and raisin, uncoated	1 bar (1 oz)	127	2	18	2	na	5	3/na	0	71	87

Food	Serving	Cal	Prot (g)	Carb (g)	Fiber (g)	Sugars (g)	Total Fat (g)	Sat/Trans Fat (g)	Chol (g)	Sod (mg)	GI
Granola bar, soft, peanut butter, uncoated	1 bar (1 oz)	119	3	18	1	na	4	1/na	0	115	87
Granola bar, soft, peanut butter and chocolate chip, uncoated	1 bar (1 oz)	121	3	17	1	na	6	2/na	0	92	87
Granola bar, soft, plain, uncoated	1 bar (1 oz)	124	2	19	1	na	5	2/na	0	78	87
Granola bar, soft, raisin, uncoated	1 bar (1.5 oz)	193	3	29	2	na	8	4/na	0	121	87
Granola bar, soft, raisin, uncoated	1 bar (1 oz)	125	2	19	1	na	5	3/na	0	79	87

Food	Serving	Cal	Prot (g)	Carb (g)	Fiber (g)	Sugars (g)	Total Fat (g)	Sat/Trans Fat (g)	Chol (mg)	Sod (mg)
CHEESES										
Cheese, Full Fat										
Cheese, blue	1 oz	100	6	1	0	t	8	5/na	21	395
Cheese, brick	1 oz	105	7	1	0	t	8	3/na	27	159
Brie	1 oz	95	6	t	0	t	8	5/na	28	178
Camembert	1 oz	85	6	t	0	t	7	4/na	20	239
Caraway	1 oz	107	7	1	0	t	8	5/na	26	196
Cheddar	1 oz	114	7	t	0	t	9	6/na	30	176
Colby	1 oz	112	6	1	0	t	9	6/na	27	171
Cream cheese	1 tbsp	51	1	t	0	t	5	3/na	16	43
Creamed cottage, large or small curd, full fat	½ cup, small curd, not packed	116	14	3	0	t	5	3/na	17	456

Food	Serving	Cal	Prot (g)	Carb (g)	Fiber (g)	Sugars (g)	Total Fat (g)	Sat/Trans Fat (g)	Chol (mg)	Sod (mg)
Creamed cottage, full fat w/fruit	½ cup, not packed	140	11	15	0	3	4	2/na	12	458
Edam	1 oz	101	7	t	0	t	8	5/na	25	274
Feta	1 oz	75	4	1	0	1	6	4/na	25	316
Fontina	1 oz	110	7	t	0	t	9	5/na	33	227
Goat, hard type	1 oz	128	9	1	0	.5	10	7/na	30	98
Goat, semisoft type	1 oz	103	6	1	0	1	8	6/na	22	146
Goat, soft type	1 oz	76	5	t	t	.5	6	4/na	13	104
Gouda	1 oz	101	7	1	0	2	8	5/na	32	232
Gruyere	1 oz	117	8	t	0	t	9	5/na	31	95
Limburger	1 oz	93	6	t	0	t	8	5/na	26	227
Low-sodium, cheddar or colby	1 oz	113	7	1	0	t	9	6/na	28	6
Monterey	1 oz	106	7	t	0	t	9	5/na	25	152
Mozzarella, low-sodium	1 cup shredded	316	31	3.5	0	1	9	12/na	61	18

Food	Serving	Cal	Prot (g)	Carb (g)	Fiber (g)	Sugars (g)	Total Fat (g)	Sat/Trans Fat (g)	Chol (mg)	Sod (mg)
Mozzarella, whole milk	1 oz	80	6	1	0	1	6	4/na	22	106
Mozzarella, whole milk, low moisture	1 oz	90	6	1	0	1	7	4/na	25	118
Muenster	1 oz	104	7	t	0	t	9	5/na	27	178
Neufchatel	1 oz	74	3	1	0	na	7	4/na	22	113
Parmesan, grated	2 tbsp	46	4	t	0	t	3	2/na	8	186
Parmesan, hard	1 oz	111	10	1	0	t	7	5/na	19	454
Port de Salut	1 oz	100	7	t	0	t	8	5/na	35	151
Provolone	1 oz	100	7	1	0	t	8	5/na	20	248
Ricotta, whole milk	½ cup	214	14	4	0	t	16	10/na	63	103
Romano	1 oz	110	9	1	0	t	8	5/na	29	340
Roquefort	1 oz	105	6	1	0	na	9	5/na	26	513
Swiss	1 oz	107	8	1	0	t	8	5/na	26	74
Cheese, Processed										
American, processed pasteurized, w/o disodium phosphate	1 oz	106	6	t	0	2	9	6/na	27	184

110

Food	Serving	Cal	Prot (g)	Carb (g)	Fiber (g)	Sugars (g)	Total Fat (g)	Sat/Trans Fat (g)	Chol (mg)	Sod (mg)
American, processed pasteurized, w/disodium phosphate	1 oz	106	6	t	0	2	9	6/na	27	405
American spread, w/o disodium phosphate	1 oz	82	5	2	0	2	6	4/na	16	381
American spread, w/disodium phosphate	1 oz	82	5	2	0	2	6	4/na	16	461
Cheddar, pasteurized process, low-sodium	1 slice	79	5	0	0	0	7	4/na	20	1
Cheese Spread	1 oz	85	5	3	0	2	6	4/na	22	420
Cheese Sauce	2 tbsp	91	4	3	t	2	7	4/na	25	541
Imitation cheese, American or cheddar, low cholesterol	1 cubic inch	70	4	0	0	t	6	1/na	3	121
Pimento processed cheese	1 oz	106	6	t	0	t	9	6/na	27	405
Swiss processed cheese	1 oz	95	7	t	0	na	7	5/na	24	193

Food	Serving	Cal	Prot (g)	Carb (g)	Fiber (g)	Sugars (g)	Total Fat (g)	Sat/Trans Fat (g)	Chol (mg)	Sod (mg)
Cheese, Reduced Fat										
Cheddar, low-fat	1 oz	98	14	1	0	0	4	2/na	12	347
Colby, low-fat	1 oz	98	14	1	0	0	4	2/na	12	347
Cottage, low-fat, 1% milk fat	½ cup	81	14	3	0	3	1	t/na	5	459
Cottage, low-fat, 2% milk fat	½ cup	102	16	4	0	0	2	1/na	9	459
Cottage, nonfat	½ cup	62	13	1	0	2	t	t/na	5	9
Cream cheese, fat-free	1 tbsp	24	3.5	1.5	0	t	t	t/na	2	136
Cream cheese, low-fat	1 tbsp	35	1.5	1	0	t	3	1.5/na	8	44
Mozzarella, nonfat	1 cup shredded	168	36	4	2	1.5	0	0/0	20	840
Mozzarella, part skim milk	1 oz	72	7	1	0	t	5	3/na	16	132
Mozzarella, part skim milk, low moisture	1 oz	79	8	1	0	t	5	3/na	15	150
Muenster, low-fat	1 slice	77	7	1	0	1	5	3/na	18	168
Ricotta, part skim	½ cup	170	14	6	0	0	10	6/na	38	154

Food	Serving	Cal	Prot (g)	Carb (g)	Fiber (g)	Sugars (g)	Total Fat (g)	Sat/Trans Fat (g)	Chol (mg)	Sod (mg)
Swiss, low-fat	1 slice	50	8	1	0	t	1.5	1/na	10	73
Swiss, processed, low-fat	1 slice	36	5	1	0	t	1	.5/na	7	300
CHICKEN										
Breast, meat only, roasted broiler or fryer	4 oz	186	35	0	0	0	4	1/0	96	84
Chicken w/skin, roasted	4 oz	272	31	0	0	0	15	4/0	100	92
Chicken, dark meat, w/skin, roasted	4 oz	288	29	0	0	0	18	5/0	104	100
Cornish game hen, meat only, roasted	½ bird	147	26	0	0	0	4	1/0	117	69
Cornish game hen, meat and skin, roasted	½ bird	335	29	0	0	0	23	6/0	169	83
Dark meat, roasted, broiler or fryer	4 oz	232	31	0	0	0	11	3/0	105	105
Dark meat, roasted, roaster	4 oz	201	26	0	0	0	10	3/0	85	107
Drumstick, meat only, roasted, broiler or fryer	4 oz	194	32	0	0	0	6	2/0	105	105

113

Food	Serving	Cal	Prot (g)	Carb (g)	Fiber (g)	Sugars (g)	Total Fat (g)	Sat/Trans Fat (g)	Chol (mg)	Sod (mg)
Drumstick, meat only, roasted, broiler or fryer	1 drumstick	76	12	0	0	0	2	1/0	41	42
Leg, meat only, roasted, broiler or fryer	1 leg	181	26	0	0	0	8	2/0	89	86
Light meat, roasted, broiler or fryer	4 oz	195	35	0	0	0	5	1/0	96	87
Light meat, roasted, roaster	4 oz	173	31	0	0	0	5	1/0	85	58
Light meat, stewed, stewer	4 oz	241	37	0	0	0	9	2/0	79	66
Wing, meat only, roasted, broiler or fryer	1 wing	43	6	0	0	0	2	t/0	18	19

Food	Serving	Cal	Prot (g)	Carb (g)	Fiber (g)	Sugars (g)	Total Fat (g)	Sat/Trans Fat (g)	Chol (g)	Sod (mg)	GI
CONDIMENTS											
Barbecue sauce	2 tbsp	53	0	13	t	9	t	t/0	0	392	is
Catsup	1 tbsp	15	t	4	t	3.5	t	t/0	0	167	55
Catsup, green	1 tbsp	20	0	5	0	4	0	0/0	0	190	55
Catsup, low-sodium	1 tbsp	15	t	4	t	3.5	t	t/0	0	3	55
Chili sauce w/salt	1 packet	6	t	1	t	t	t	t/0	0	80	is
Chili sauce, low-sodium	1 tbsp	18	t	5	t	3	t	t/0	1	3	is
Cocktail sauce (Del Monte)	2 tbsp	50	t	12	na	11	0	0/0	0	455	is
Enchilada sauce (Ortega)	2 tbsp	15	t	1	t	t	t	t/0	0	77	is
Horseradish	1 tbsp	7	t	2	t	na	t	t/0	0	47	is
Hot pepper sauce	¼ tsp	0	t	t	0	na	0	0/0	0	32	is
Mustard (Grey Poupon)	1 tbsp	15	0	0	0	na	0	0/0	0	360	is
Mustard, yellow	1 tbsp	10	t	1	t	na	t	t/0	0	168	is
Picante sauce (Ortega)	2 tbsp	10	t	2	0	t	t	t/0	0	252	is

115

Food	Serving	Cal	Prot (g)	Carb (g)	Fiber (g)	Sugars (g)	Total Fat (g)	Sat/Trans Fat (g)	Chol (g)	Sod (mg)	GI
Picante sauce, medium (La Victoria)	2 tbsp	8	t	1	t	1	t	na/na	0	150	is
Picante sauce, mild (La Victoria)	2 tbsp	8	t	1	t	1	t	na/na	0	179	is
Salsa	2 tbsp	9	t	2	t	na	t	t/0	0	139	is
Salsa, black bean and corn	2 tbsp	16	1	3	.5	1	0	0/0	0	125	is
Salsa, Chunky Chili Dip (La Victoria)	2 tbsp	9	t	2	t	na	t	na/na	na	148	is
Salsa, green chili, mild (La Victoria)	2 tbsp	8	t	1	t	t	t	na/na	na	172	is
Salsa, green jalapena (La Victoria)	2 tbsp	10	t	1	t	t	t	na/na	0	180	is
Salsa Ranchero, hot (La Victoria)	2 tbsp	9	t	2	t	1	t	na/na	0	169	is
Salsa, red jalapena (La Victoria)	2 tbsp	12	t	2	t	1	t	t/na	0	146	is
Salsa, Thick 'N Chunky, hot (La Victoria)	2 tbsp	8	t	1	t	1	t	na/na	0	131	is
Salsa, Thick 'N Chunky, medium (La Victoria)	2 tbsp	8	t	1	t	1	t	t/0	0	158	is

Food	Serving	Cal	Prot (g)	Carb (g)	Fiber (g)	Sugars (g)	Total Fat (g)	Sat/Trans Fat (g)	Chol (g)	Sod (mg)	GI
Salsa, Thick 'N Chunky, mild (La Victoria)	2 tbsp	8	t	1	t	1	t	na/na	0	156	is
Spaghetti/marinara sauce	½ cup	71	2	10	2	na	3	t/0	0	515	is
Tabasco sauce	1 tsp	1	t	t	0	na	t	t/0	0	30	is
Taco sauce, green, mild (La Victoria)	2 tbsp	9	t	2	t	1	t	na/na	0	190	is
Taco sauce, green, mild (La Victoria)	2 tbsp	9	t	2	t	1	t	na/na	0	190	is
Taco sauce, red, medium (La Victoria)	2 tbsp	13	t	3	t	2	t	t/0	0	210	is
Taco sauce, red, mild (La Victoria)	2 tbsp	13	t	3	t	2	t	na/na	0	210	is
Tartar sauce, low-calorie	1 tbsp	31	t	2	na	na	2.5	t/0	3	82	is
Teriyaki sauce, generic	2 tbsp	30	2	6	0	na	0	0/0	0	1380	is
Teriyaki sauce (Kikkoman)	2 tbsp	30	2	4	0	4	0	0/0	0	610	is
Teriyaki sauce (Nestlé)	2 tbsp	42	t	7	0	6	1	t/0	0	319	is

117

Food	Serving	Cal	Prot (g)	Carb (g)	Fiber (g)	Sugars (g)	Total Fat (g)	Sat/Trans Fat (g)	Chol (g)	Sod (mg)	GI
Vinegar	1 tbsp	1	0	t	0	t	t	0/0	0	0	5
Worcestershire sauce	1 tsp	0	0	0	0	0	0	0/0	0	60	is
CRACKERS											
Butter-type	1 serving	79	1	10	t	1	4	1/na	0	124	na
Cheese, regular	1 cup, bite size	312	6	36	1.5	t	16	6/na	8	617	54
Cheese, sandwich-type, w/peanut butter filling	4 crackers	129	3	15	1	2	7	1/na	1	185	na
Crispbread, rye (including Wasa crispbread)	2 crackers	74	2	16	3	t	t	t/na	0	52	63
Crispbread, rye, large (triple cracker)	1 cracker	92	2	21	4	t	t	t/na	0	66	63
Flatbread, Norwegian	3 crackers	63	1	14	3	na	t	t/na	0	45	79
French onion snack	1 serving	128	2	23	1	2	3	1/na	1	275	na

Food	Serving	Cal	Prot (g)	Carb (g)	Fiber (g)	Sugars (g)	Total Fat (g)	Sat/Trans Fat (g)	Chol (g)	Sod (mg)	GI
Italian ranch snack	1 serving	128	2	23	1	2	3	1/na	1	311	na
Matzo, plain	1 matzo	111	3	23	1	t	t	t/na	0	1	70
Matzo, whole wheat	1 matzo	98	4	22	3	na	t	t/na	0	1	40
Melba toast, rye	4 toasts	76	2	15	2	na	1	t/na	0	180	70
Melba toast, wheat	4 toasts	76	3	15	2	na	t	t/na	0	168	70
Oyster	½ cup	98	2	16	1	na	3	1/na	0	293	74
Oyster, low-salt	½ cup	98	2	16	1	na	3	1/na	0	143	74
Rye, sandwich-type, w/peanut butter filling	4 crackers	135	3	17	1	na	6	2	3	292	na
Rye wafers, plain	2 wafers	74	2	18	5	1	t	t/na	0	174	na
Rye wafers, seasoned, large (triple cracker)	1 wafer	84	2	16	5	na	2	t/na	0	195	na
Salsa snack	1 serving	128	2	23	1	2	3	1/na	1	321	na
Saltines	1 serving	51	1	8.5	t	t	1	t/t	0	129	74
Saltines, fat-free, low-sodium	4 crackers	79	2	16.5	.5	t	t	t/t	0	127	74

Food	Serving	Cal	Prot (g)	Carb (g)	Fiber (g)	Sugars (g)	Total Fat (g)	Sat/Trans Fat (g)	Chol (g)	Sod (mg)	GI
Snack-type, sandwich-type w/cheese filling	4 crackers	134	3	17	.5	1	5	2/na	1	392	na
Wheat, sandwich-type, w/cheese filling	4 crackers	139	3	16	1	na	7	1/na	2	256	na
Wheat, sandwich-type, w/peanut butter filling	4 crackers	139	4	15	1	na	7	1/na	0	226	na
Wheat, thin-type	1 serving	136	2	20	1	3	6	1/na	0	168	na
Whole-wheat crackers	4 crackers	72	1	10	2	na	3	t/na	0	104	na
Whole-wheat crackers, low-salt	4 crackers	72	1	10	2	na	3	t/na	0	40	na
DIABETIC SUPPORT PRODUCTS											
Boost Diabetic (Novartis)	8 oz	250	14	20	3.5	na	11.7	na/na	na	260	na
Boost Glucose Control (Novartis)	8 oz	190	16	16	3	na	3	na/na	na	250	na
Choice dm Bar (Mead Johnson Nutritionals)	1 bar	140	6	19	3	9	4.5	na/na	na	na	na
Choice dm Crispy Bar (Mead Johnson Nutritionals)	1 bar	120	4	21	1	5	2.5	na/na	na	na	na

120

Food	Serving	Cal	Prot (g)	Carb (g)	Fiber (g)	Sugars (g)	Total Fat (g)	Sat/Trans Fat (g)	Chol (g)	Sod (mg)	GI
Dietsource Sorbet (Novartis)	3 fl oz	20	0	5	na	na	0	0/0	0	30	na
Dietsource Sugar-Free Gelatin Mix (Novartis)	4 oz serving (dry mix)	10	2	1	0	0	0/0	0/0	0	0	na
Dietsource Sugar-Free Pudding Mix, vanilla (Novartis)	4 oz serving (12 g dry mix w/4 oz skim milk)	80	4	16	na	0	0	0/0	0	190	na
Extend Diabetes Snack Bar, chocolate chip crunch (Clinical Product, Ltd.)	1 bar	150	3	31	1	10	3	1.5/0	0	80	na
Extend Diabetes Snack Bar, low-carb formula, chocolate delight (Clinical Product, Ltd.)	1 bar	140	11	21	5	0	3	1.5/0	0	150	na
Glucerna Meal Bar (Abbott Laboratories)	1 bar	220	10	34	2	11	7	3.5/0	0	180	na

Food	Serving	Cal	Prot (g)	Carb (g)	Fiber (g)	Sugars (g)	Total Fat (g)	Sat/Trans Fat (g)	Chol (g)	Sod (mg)	GI
Glucerna Shakes (Abbott Laboratories)	8 oz	220	10	29	4	7	8.5	1/0	.5	210	31
Glucerna Snack Bars (Abbott Laboratories)	1 bar	150	6	25	1	3	4	3/0	0	150	na
GlucoBurst Diabetic Drink	8 oz	190	10	19	3	0	8.5	.5/0	na	na	na
GlucoBurst Glucose Gel	1 pouch (1.3 oz)	70	0	16	0	15	0	0/0	0	30	na
Gluco-O-Bar (APIC, USA, Inc.)	1 bar	130	7	21	0	1	2.5	na/na	na	na	na
Nite Bite Timed-Release Glucose Bar (ICN Pharmaceuticals, Inc.)	1 bar	100	3	15	0	10	3.5	na/na	na	na	na
Nutrisource Quick Reduced Calorie Custard (Novartis)	4 oz (prepared w/ skim milk)	60	5	10	na	na	0	0/0	0	125	na
Resource Diabetishield (Novartis)	8 oz	150	7	30	na	na	0	0/0	0	<80	16
Resource No Sugar Added Health Shake, vanilla (Novartis)	4 fl oz	200	8	22	na	na	9	2.5/na	10	115	na

Food	Serving	Cal	Prot (g)	Carb (g)	Fiber (g)	Sugars (g)	Total Fat (g)	Sat/Trans Fat (g)	Chol (mg)	Sod (mg)
EGGS										
Egg, fried	1 large	92	6	1	0	0	7	2/0	211	162
Egg, scrambled	1 large	101	7	1	0	0	7	2/0	215	171
Egg substitute, liquid	¼ cup	53	8	t	0	0	2	t/0	1	111
Egg white	2 large	33	7	t	0	0	0	0/0	0	108
Egg white, dried powder	1 tbsp	53	12	1	0	0	t	0/0	0	173
Egg, whole, fresh	1 extra large	86	7	1	0	0	6	2/0	246	73
Egg, whole, fresh	1 jumbo	97	8	1	0	0	6.5	2/0	276	82
Egg, whole, fresh	1 large	75	6	1	0	0	5	1.5/0	213	63
Egg, whole, fresh	1 medium	66	5.5	.5	0	0	4	1/0	187	55
Egg, whole, fresh	1 small	55	5	t	0	0	4	1/0	157	47
Egg, whole, hard-boiled	1 large	78	6	t	0	0	5	2/0	212	62
Egg, whole, poached	1 large	75	6	t	0	0	5	2/0	212	140
Omelet	1 large	93	6	1	0	0	7	2/0	214	165

Food	Serving	Cal	Prot (g)	Carb (g)	Fiber (g)	Sugars (g)	Total Fat (g)	Sat/Trans Fat (g)	Chol (g)	Sod (mg)	GI
ENTREES AND COMBINATION FOODS											
Canned											
Beef ravioli in tomato and meat sauce	1 serving	229	8	37	4	5	5	2/t	15	1,174	60
Beef ravioli in tomato and meat sauce, mini ravioli	1 serving	239	9	41	3	5	5	2/t	18	1,197	60
Beef stew	1 serving	218	11	16	4	2	12	5/na	37	947	66
Chicken and dumplings, canned	1 serving	218	15	23	3	2	7	2/na	36	946	na
Chow mein, no noodles or rice	2 cups	160	16	12	6	4	7	3/na	40	2,380	47–55
Corned beef hash	1 cup	387	21	22	3	1	24	10/na	76	1,003	na
Macaroni w/beef in tomato sauce	1 serving	184	8	31	3	5	3	1/t	17	799	na
Macaroni and cheese	1 serving	199	8	29	3	2	5	3/na	8	1,058	64
Roast beef hash	1 cup	385	21	23	4	1	24	10/na	73	793	na
Spaghetti and meatballs in tomato sauce	1 serving	250	9	34	2	6	9	4/t	22	941	52

Food	Serving	Cal	Prot (g)	Carb (g)	Fiber (g)	Sugars (g)	Total Fat (g)	Sat/Trans Fat (g)	Chol (g)	Sod (mg)	GI
Frozen											
Beef macaroni	1 serving	211	14	33	5	9	2	1/na	14	444	na
Beef pot pie	1 serving	449	13	44	2	na	24	9/na	38	737	45
Beef Pot Roast (Lean Cuisine)	1 serving	184	13	21	3	4	5.5	1/t	20	768	na
Beef strips w/ Oriental-style vegetables	1 serving	433	26	71	na	na	5	na/na	na	1,584	na
Beef stroganoff and noodles w/carrots and peas	1 serving	600	30	59	4	6	27	11/6	70	1,141	na
Chicken Alfredo with fettucini and vegetables	1 serving	373	19	33	4	na	18	7/na	57	588	52
Chicken cordon bleu, filled w/cheese and ham	1 serving	344	26	15	na	na	21	6/na	81	754	na
Chicken Enchilada Dinner (Weight Watchers Smart Ones)	1 serving	311	14	45	3	33	8	3.5/t	33	727	na
Chicken Enchilada Dinner (Healthy Choice)	1 meal	352	12	58	5	2	8	3/t	35	573	na

125

Food	Serving	Cal	Prot (g)	Carb (g)	Fiber (g)	Sugars (g)	Total Fat (g)	Sat/Trans Fat (g)	Chol (g)	Sod (mg)	GI
Chicken enchilada and Mexican-style rice w/Monterey jack cheese sauce	1 serving	376	12	48	5	na	15	3/na	25	1,002	na
Chicken fajita	1 serving	129	8	17	na	na	3	1/t	13	350	42
Chicken Mesquite BBQ Dinner (Healthy Choice)	1 meal	277	17	42	7	14	4	1/0	33	447	na
Chicken pot pie	1 serving	484	13	43	2	8	29	12/na	41	857	na
Chicken Teriyaki Dinner (Healthy Choice)	1 meal	250	16	36	9	14	5	1.5/0	22	596	na
Chicken and Vegetables (Lean Cuisine)	1 serving	232	20	26	4	5	5	2/t	30	633	na
Creamed chipped beef	1 serving	175	10	7	na	na	12	5/t	44	621	na
Dinner-type meal (TV), generic, frozen	1 meal (16 oz)	512	27	54	6	9	21	7/na	59	1,402	na
Fried chicken w/mashed potatoes and corn in sauce	1 serving	470	21	35	2	3	27	9/1	89	1,500	na
Escalloped chicken and noodles	1 serving	419	17	31	na	na	25	7/na	76	1,211	na
Italian sausage lasagna	1 serving	456	21	40	3	na	24	8/na	48	903	na

Food	Serving	Cal	Prot (g)	Carb (g)	Fiber (g)	Sugars (g)	Total Fat (g)	Sat/Trans Fat (g)	Chol (g)	Sod (mg)	GI
Lasagna w/meat and sauce	1 serving	377	19	26	3	na	11	5/na	41	735	na
Lasagna w/meat and sauce, low-fat	1 serving	312	21	42	4	2	7	3/na	22	559	na
Macaroni and Beef in Tomato Sauce (Lean Cuisine)	1 serving	258	17	37	5	11	5	2/t	17	569	na
Meat loaf dinner w/tomato sauce, mashed potatoes and carrots in seasoned sauce	1 serving	612	29	34	6	12	40	15/na	113	1,943	na
Mexican-style dinner w/tamales, beef enchiladas and chili sauce, beans and rice	1 serving	508	14	68	8	na	20	7/na	26	1,812	na
Oriental Beef with Vegetables and Rice (Lean Cuisine)	1 serving	189	13	28	4	8	3	1/t	23	536	na
Roasted chicken w/garlic sauce, pasta and vegetable medley	1 serving	214	17	22	4	na	7	1/na	28	467	na
Salisbury steak in gravy, w/macaroni and cheese	1 serving	386	23	26	na	na	21	8/na	63	1,015	na
Salisbury steak in gravy, w/ mashed potatoes and corn in seasoned sauce	1 serving	782	27	47	7	7	54	21/na	131	2,195	na

127

Food	Serving	Cal	Prot (g)	Carb (g)	Fiber (g)	Sugars (g)	Total Fat (g)	Sat/Trans Fat (g)	Chol (g)	Sod (mg)	GI
Sliced beef meal, w/gravy, mashed potatoes and peas in seasoned sauce	1 serving	270	26	19	4	12	10	4/na	71	742	na
Spaghetti with Meatballs and Sauce (Lean Cuisine)	1 serving	250	18	33	4	7	5	2/t	24	568	na
Spaghetti with Meat Sauce (Lean Cuisine)	1 serving	284	14	49	5	8	4	1/t	13	548	na
Stuffed Cabbage with Meat (Lean Cuisine)	1 serving	196	11	24	4	6	6	2/t	13	710	na
Stuffed peppers w/beef, in tomato sauce	1 serving	189	8	21	5	na	8	3/.5	22	579	na
Swedish Meatballs (Lean Cuisine)	1 serving	273	22	31	3	5	7	3/t	49	614	na
Tuna noodle casserole	1 cup	259	13	34	2	1	8	2/na	42	1,043	na
Turkey and gravy w/dressing and broccoli	1 serving	504	31	52	0	11	19	9/na	79	2,037	na
Turkey and gravy w/dressing meal, w/mashed potatoes and corn in seasoned sauce	1 serving	280	14	34	3	7	10	3/na	52	1,061	na

Food	Serving	Cal	Prot (g)	Carb (g)	Fiber (g)	Sugars (g)	Total Fat (g)	Sat/Trans Fat (g)	Chol (g)	Sod (mg)	GI
Turkey Medallions dinner (Weight Watchers Smart Ones)	1 serving	214	13	38	3	1	1	.5/na	56	548	na
Turkey pot pie	1 serving	699	26	70	4	na	35	11/na	64	1,390	na
Veal parmigiana meal w/tomato sauce, mashed potatoes and peas in seasoned sauce	1 serving	362	13	35	7	15	19	6/na	26	964	na
FAST FOOD/SALADS											
Arby's											
Chicken Club Salad	1 serving	503	32	31	3	3	26	8/2	208	1,235	na
Martha's Vineyard Salad	1 serving	276	26	24	4	16	8	4/0	72	454	na
Santa Fe Salad	1 serving	210	30	41	6	5	231	8/2	59	1,231	na
Santa Fe Salad w/Grilled Chicken	1 serving	306	30	20	5	7	11	6/1	78	621	na
Burger King											
Tendergrill Chicken Garden Salad	1 serving	240	33	8	4	3	9	3.5/0	80	720	na
Tendercrisp Chicken Garden Salad	1 serving	400	22	32	5	5	21	7/3.5	70	1,170	na

129

Food	Serving	Cal	Prot (g)	Carb (g)	Fiber (g)	Sugars (g)	Total Fat (g)	Sat/Trans Fat (g)	Chol (g)	Sod (mg)	GI
Chick-Fil-A											
Chargrilled Chicken Garden Salad	1 serving	180	22	9	3	6	6	3/0	65	620	na
Chicken Strips Salad	1 serving	400	34	21	4	7	20	6/0	80	1,070	na
Southwest Chargrilled Salad	1 serving	240	25	17	5	6	8	3.5/0	60	770	na
Dairy Queen											
Grilled Chicken Salad w/fat-free Italian dressing	1 serving	240	26	12	4	7	10	5/0	65	950	na
Crispy Chicken Salad	1 serving	350	21	21	6	9	20	6/2.5	40	620	na
Jack in the Box											
Asian Chicken Salad	1 serving	140	14	19	5	13	10	0/0	25	470	na
Chicken Club Salad	1 serving	300	27	13	4	7	15	6/0	65	880	na
Southwest Chicken Salad	1 serving	300	24	29	78	8	11	1.5/0	550	860	na
McDonald's											
Southwest Salad w/Grilled Chicken	1 serving	320	30	30	7	11	9	3/0	70	970	na
Southwest Salad w/Crispy Chicken	1 serving	400	25	41	7	10	16	4/1.5	50	1,110	na

Food	Serving	Cal	Prot (g)	Carb (g)	Fiber (g)	Sugars (g)	Total Fat (g)	Sat/Trans Fat (g)	Chol (g)	Sod (mg)	GI
Southwest Salad w/o chicken	1 serving	140	6	20	6	5	4.5	2/0	10	150	na
Asian Salad w/Grilled Chicken	1 serving	300	32	23	5	12	10	1/0	65	890	na
Asian Salad w/Crispy Chicken	1 serving	380	27	33	5	12	17	2.5/1.5	45	1,030	na
Asian Salad w/o chicken	1 serving	150	8	15	5	9	7	.5/0	0	35	na
Bacon Ranch Salad w/Grilled Chicken	1 serving	260	33	12	3	5	9	4/0	90	1,010	na
Bacon Ranch Salad w/Crispy Chicken	1 serving	350	28	23	3	4	16	5/1.5	70	1,150	na
Bacon Ranch Salad w/o chicken	1 serving	140	9	10	3	4	7	3.5/0	25	300	na
Caesar Salad w/Grilled Chicken	1 serving	220	30	12	3	5	6	3/0	75	890	na
Caesar Salad w/Crispy Chicken	1 serving	300	25	22	3	4	13	4/1.5	55	1,020	na
Caesar Salad w/o chicken	1 serving	90	7	9	3	4	4	2.5/0	10	180	na
Subway											
Grilled Chicken & Baby Spinach	1 serving	140	20	11	4	4	3	1/0	50	450	na
Subway Club Turkey	1 serving	160	18	15	4	7	4	1.5/0	35	880	na

Food	Serving	Cal	Prot (g)	Carb (g)	Fiber (g)	Sugars (g)	Total Fat (g)	Sat/Trans Fat (g)	Chol (g)	Sod (mg)	GI
Tuna (w/cheese)	1 serving	360	16	12	4	5	29	6/.5	45	600	na
Veggie Delite	1 serving	60	3	12	4	5	1	0/0	0	90	na
Wendy's											
Caesar Chicken Salad	1 serving	190	27	9	4	4	5	2.5/0	70	620	na
Mandarin Chicken Salad	1 serving	170	23	18	3	13	2	2.5/0	60	480	na
Chicken BLT Salad	1 serving	340	35	17	4	6	18	9/0	100	980	na
Southwest Taco Salad	1 serving	440	30	32	9	10	22	12/1	80	1,100	na
FAST FOOD/SANDWICHES & WRAPS											
Burger King											
BK Veggie Burger, w/o mayo	1 serving	340	23	46	7	8	8	1/0	0	1,030	na
Original Chicken Sandwich, w/o mayo	1 serving	450	23	52	4	5	17	4/2	50	1,250	na
Tendergrill™ Chicken Sandwich, w/o sauce	1 serving	400	36	49	4	7	7	1.5/0	70	1,090	na

Food	Serving	Cal	Prot (g)	Carb (g)	Fiber (g)	Sugars (g)	Total Fat (g)	Sat/Trans Fat (g)	Chol (g)	Sod (mg)	GI
Chick-Fil-A											
Chargrilled	1 serving	270	28	33	3	7	3.5	1/0	65	940	na
Chicken Sandwich, w/o butter	1 serving	380	28	37	1	5	13	3/0	60	1,290	na
Chargrilled Chicken Deluxe Sandwich, w/o Butter	1 serving	420	28	39	2	5	16	3.5/0	60	1,300	na
Chargrilled Chicken Cool Wrap®	1 serving	390	29	54	3	7	7	3/0	65	1,020	na
Chicken Caesar Wrap®	1 serving	460	36	52	3	5	10	6/0	80	1,350	na
Spicy Chicken Cool Wrap®	1 serving	380	30	52	3	5	6	3/0	60	1,090	na
Dairy Queen											
Grilled Chicken Sandwich	1 serving	340	21	50	5	8	16	6/2	40	1,100	na
Jack in the Box											
Chicken Fajita Pita	1 serving	300	23	31	3	4	10	4.5/0	65	880	na
Chicken Sandwich	1 serving	400	15	38	2	4	21	4.5/2.5	35	730	na
Southwest Chicken Pita	1 serving	230	18	34	3	3	3.5	1/0	40	790	na

133

Food	Serving	Cal	Prot (g)	Carb (g)	Fiber (g)	Sugars (g)	Total Fat (g)	Sat/Trans Fat (g)	Chol (g)	Sod (mg)	GI
Subway (sandwiches with 6 grams of fat or less)											
Ham	1 serving	290	18	47	4	8	5	1.5/0	25	1,280	na
Oven Roasted Chicken Breast	1 serving	330	24	48	5	9	5	1.5/0	45	1,020	na
Roast Beef	1 serving	290	19	45	4	8	5	2/0	20	920	na
Subway Club®	1 serving	320	24	47	4	8	6	2/0	35	1,310	na
Sweet Onion Teriyaki	1 serving	370	26	59	4	19	5	1.5/0	50	1,220	na
Turkey Breast	1 serving	280	18	46	4	7	4.5	1.5/0	20	1,020	na
Turkey Breast & Ham	1 serving	290	20	47	4	8	5	1.5/0	25	1,250	na
Veggie Delite	1 serving	230	9	44	4	7	3	1/0	0	520	na
Wendy's											
Ultimate Chicken Grill Sandwich	1 serving	370	33	44	2	10	8	1.5/0	60	1,070	na
FAST FOOD/SOUPS											
Chick-Fil-A											
Hearty Breast of Chicken Soup	1 cup	140	8	18	1	2	3.5	1/0	25	900	na

134

Food	Serving	Cal	Prot (g)	Carb (g)	Fiber (g)	Sugars (g)	Total Fat (g)	Sat/Trans Fat (g)	Chol (g)	Sod (mg)	GI
Subway											
Brown and Wild Rice w/Chicken	10 oz bowl	220	6	26	1	3	11	3.5/0	50	1,170	na
Chili con Carne	10 oz bowl	340	20	35	10	7	11	5/0	60	1,100	na
Minestrone	10 oz bowl	90	4	17	4	4	.5	0/0	0	910	na
Roasted Chicken Noodle	10 oz bowl	90	7	12	1	2	1.5	.5/0	20	1,130	na
Spanish Style Chicken w/Rice	10 oz bowl	110	7	16	1	1	2	0/0	5	980	na
Tomato Garden Vegetable w/Rotini	10 oz bowl	100	3	20	3	8	.5	0/0	40	1,040	na
Vegetable Beef	10 oz bowl	100	5	17	3	5	1	.5/0	5	1,060	na
Wendy's											
Chili, small	8 oz	227	17	23	5	6	6	2.5/0	35	780	na
Chili, large	12 oz	340	25	35	8	9	9	3.5/.5	55	1,170	na
FAST FOOD/MEXICAN/VARIOUS											
Bean Burrito (Taco Bell)	1 burrito	404	16	55	8	5	14	5/na	18	1,216	na
Burrito w/beans	1 burrito	224	7	36	na	na	7	3/na	2	493	na
Burrito w/beans and cheese	1 burrito	189	8	27	na	na	6	3/na	14	583	na

135

Food	Serving	Cal	Prot (g)	Carb (g)	Fiber (g)	Sugars (g)	Total Fat (g)	Sat/Trans Fat (g)	Chol (g)	Sod (mg)	GI
Burrito w/beans and chili peppers	1 burrito	206	8	29	na	na	7	4/na	16	522	na
Burrito w/beans and meat	1 burrito	254	11	33	na	na	9	4/na	24	668	na
Burrito w/beans, cheese, and beef	1 burrito	165	7	20	na	na	7	3.5/na	62	495	na
Burrito w/beans, cheese, and chili peppers	1 burrito	331	17	43	na	na	11	6/na	79	1,030	na
Burrito w/beef	1 burrito	262	13	29	na	na	10	5/na	32	746	na
Burrito w/beef and chili peppers	1 burrito	213	11	25	na	na	8	4/na	27	558	na
Burrito w/beef, cheese, and chili peppers	1 burrito	316	20	32	na	na	12	5/na	85	1,046	na
Burrito Supreme w/beef (Taco Bell)	1 burrito	469	20	52	8	6	20	8/na	40	1,424	na
Burrito Supreme w/chicken (Taco Bell)	1 burrito	444	24	51	6	3	16	6/na	52	1,399	na
Burrito Supreme w/steak (Taco Bell)	1 burrito	454	23	50	6	2	18	7/na	52	1,324	na
Chimichanga w/beef	1 chimi-changa	425	20	43	na	na	29	8.5/na	9	910	na

Food	Serving	Cal	Prot (g)	Carb (g)	Fiber (g)	Sugars (g)	Total Fat (g)	Sat/Trans Fat (g)	Chol (g)	Sod (mg)	GI
Chimichanga w/beef and cheese	1 chimi-changa	443	20	39	na	na	23	11/na	51	957	na
Chimichanga w/beef and red chili peppers	1 chimi-changa	424	18	46	na	na	19	8/na	10	1,169	na
Chimichanga w/beef, cheese, and red chili peppers	1 chimi-changa	364	15	38	na	na	18	8/na	50	895	na
Enchilada w/cheese	1 enchilada	319	10	28	na	na	19	11/na	44	784	na
Enchilada w/cheese and beef	1 enchilada	323	12	30	na	na	18	9/na	40	1,319	na
Enchilada w/cheese, beef, and beans	1 enchilada	344	18	34	na	na	16	8/na	50	1,251	na
Frijoles w/beans	1 cup	225	11	29	na	na	8	4/na	37	882	na
Taco	1 taco, small	369	21	27	na	na	21	11/na	56	802	na

137

Food	Serving	Cal	Prot (g)	Carb (g)	Fiber (g)	Sugars (g)	Total Fat (g)	Sat/Trans Fat (g)	Chol (g)	Sod (mg)	GI
Taco	1 taco, large	568	32	41	na	na	32	17/na	87	1,233	na
Taco (Original Taco w/Beef – Taco Bell)	1 taco	184	8	14	3	1	11	4/na	24	349	na
Taco salad	2 cups	372	18	31	na	na	20	9/na	58	1,016	na
Taco salad w/chili con carne	2 cups	386	23	35	na	na	17.5	8/na	7	1,180	na
Taco, soft w/beef (Taco Bell)	1 taco	217	12	20	3	2	10	4	28	626	na
Taco, soft w/chicken (Taco Bell)	1 taco	200	14	19	2	1	7	3/na	37	600	na
Taco, soft w/steak (Taco Bell)	1 taco	286	15	22	2	1	15	4/na	39	700	na
Tostada w/beans and cheese	1 tostada	223	10	27	na	na	10	5/na	30	543	na
Tostada w/beans, beef, and cheese	1 tostada	333	16	30	na	na	17	11/na	74	871	na
Tostada w/beef and cheese	1 tostada	315	19	23	na	na	16	10/na	41	897	na
FATS AND OILS											
Butter											
Butter, light, stick w/salt	1 oz (28 grams)	140	1	0	0	0	15.5	10/0	30	126	0

138

Food	Serving	Cal	Prot (g)	Carb (g)	Fiber (g)	Sugars (g)	Total Fat (g)	Sat/Trans Fat (g)	Chol (g)	Sod (mg)	GI
Butter, light, stick w/o salt	1 oz (28 grams)	140	1	0	0	0	15.5	10/0	30	10	0
Butter, whipped, w/salt	1 pat (1"sq×1/3" high)	27	t	0	0	0	3	2/0	8	31	0
Butter, w/o salt	1 pat (1"sq×1/3" high)	36	t	0	0	0	4	3/0	11	1	0
Butter, w/salt	1 pat (1"sq×1/3" high)	36	t	0	0	0	4	3	11	41	0
Margarine											
Fleischmann's Light Margarine	1 tbsp	40	0	0	0	0	4.5	0/0	0	90	0
Margarine, 80% fat, stick, includes regular and hydrogenated corn and soybean oils	1 tbsp	99	0	0	0	0	11	2/3	0	92	0
Margarine, 70% vegetable oil spread, soybean and soybean (hydrogenated)	1 tbsp	87	0	0	0	0	10	2/3	0	98	0

Food	Serving	Cal	Prot (g)	Carb (g)	Fiber (g)	Sugars (g)	Total Fat (g)	Sat/Trans Fat (g)	Chol (g)	Sod (mg)	GI
Margarine, regular, hard, corn (hydrogenated)	1 tsp	34	t	0	0	0	4	1/na	0	44	0
Margarine, regular, hard, safflower and soybean (hydrogenated and regular) and cottonseed (hydrogenated)	1 tsp	34	t	0	0	0	4	1/na	0	44	0
Margarine, regular, hard, safflower and soybean (hydrogenated)	1 tsp	34	t	0	0	0	4	1/na	0	44	0
Margarine, regular, hard, safflower and soybean (hydrogenated) and cottonseed (hydrogenated)	1 tsp	34	t	0	0	0	4	1/na	0	44	0
Margarine, regular, hard, soybean (hydrogenated and regular)	1 tsp	34	t	0	0	0	4	1/na	0	44	0
Margarine, regular, hard, soybean (hydrogenated)	1 tsp	34	t	0	0	0	4	1/na	0	44	0
Margarine, regular, liquid, soybean (hydrogenated and regular) and cottonseed	1 tsp	34	t	0	0	0	4	1/na	0	37	0
Margarine, regular, unspecified oils, w/salt	1 tsp	34	t	0	0	0	4	1/na	0	44	0

Food	Serving	Cal	Prot (g)	Carb (g)	Fiber (g)	Sugars (g)	Total Fat (g)	°Sat/Trans Fat (g)	Chol (g)	Sod (mg)	GI
Margarine, regular, unspecified oils, w/o salt	1 tsp	34	t	0	0	0	4	1/na	0	0	0
Margarine, soft, corn (hydrogenated and regular)	1 tsp	34	t	0	0	0	4	1/na	0	51	0
Margarine, soft, safflower (hydrogenated and regular)	1 tsp	34	t	0	0	0	4	t/na	0	51	0
Margarine, soft, soybean (hydrogenated and regular), w/salt	1 tsp	34	t	0	0	0	4	1/na	0	51	0
Margarine, regular, hard, coconut (hydrogenated and regular) and safflower and palm (hydrogenated)	1 tsp	34	t	0	0	0	4	3/na	0	44	0
Margarine, regular, hard, corn (hydrogenated and regular)	1 tsp	34	t	0	0	0	4	1/na	0	44	0
Margarine, regular, hard, corn (hydrogenated)	1 tsp	34	t	0	0	0	4	1/na	0	44	0
Margarine, regular, hard, corn and soybean (hydrogenated) and cottonseed (hydrogenated), w/salt	1 tsp	34	t	0	0	0	4	1/na	0	44	0

Food	Serving	Cal	Prot (g)	Carb (g)	Fiber (g)	Sugars (g)	Total Fat (g)	Sat/Trans Fat (g)	Chol (g)	Sod (mg)	GI
Margarine, regular, hard, corn and soybean (hydrogenated) and cottonseed (hydrogenated), w/o salt	1 tsp	34	t	0	0	0	4	1/na	0	0	0
Margarine, soft, soybean (hydrogenated) and safflower	1 tsp	34	t	0	0	0	4	1/na	0	51	0
Margarine-butter blend, 60% corn oil margarine and 40% butter	1 tsp	34	t	t	0	0	4	1/na	4	42	0
Margarine-like spread approx. 40% fat, corn (hydrogenated and regular)	1 tsp	17	t	t	0	0	2	t/na	0	46	0
Margarine-like spread approx. 40% fat, soybean (hydrogenated)	1 tsp	17	t	t	0	0	2	t/na	0	46	0
Margarine-like spread approx. 40% fat, unspecified oils	1 tsp	17	t	t	0	0	2	t/na	0	46	0
Margarine-like spread approx. 60% fat, stick, soybean (hydrogenated and regular)	1 tsp	26	t	0	0	0	3	1/na	0	48	0

Food	Serving	Cal	Prot (g)	Carb (g)	Fiber (g)	Sugars (g)	Total Fat (g)	Sat/Trans Fat (g)	Chol (g)	Sod (mg)	GI
Margarine-like spread approx. 60% fat, tub, unspecified oils	1 tsp	26	t	0	0	0	3	1/na	0	48	0
Parkay Light Stick	1 tbsp	50	0	0	0	0	5	1/na	0	75	0
Promise Buttery Light	1 tbsp	50	0	0	0	0	6	1.5/0	0	85	0
Sprays and Pumps											
I Can't Believe It's Not Butter Spray	5 sprays	0	0	0	0	0	0	0/0	0	0	0
Pam and similar vegetable sprays	1 spray	7	na	0	na	na	1	t/0	na	na	0
Tubs and Squeeze Bottles											
Benecol Spread	1 tbsp	80	0	0	0	0	9	1/0	0	110	0
Benecol Light Spread	1 tbsp	45	0	0	0	0	5	.5/0	0	110	0
Blue Bonnet Home Style Spread	1 tbsp	60	0	0	0	0	7	1.5/0	0	110	0
Brummel & Brown Spread with Yogurt	1 tbsp	45	0	0	0	0	5	1/0	0	0	0
Canoleo Margarine	1 tbsp	100	0	0	0	0	11	1/0	0	120	0
Earth Balance Natural Buttery Spread	1 tbsp	100	0	0	0	0	11	1/0	0	120	0

143

Food	Serving	Cal	Prot (g)	Carb (g)	Fiber (g)	Sugars (g)	Total Fat (g)	Sat/Trans Fat (g)	Chol (g)	Sod (mg)	GI
Fleischmann's Light Margarine	1 tbsp	40	0	0	0	0	4.5	0/0	0	90	0
Fleischmann's Original Spread	1 tbsp	80	0	0	0	0	8	1.5/0	0	75	0
Fleischmann's Premium Spread with Olive Oil	1 tbsp	70	0	0	0	0	8	1.5/0	0	95	0
Fleischmann's Unsalted Spread	1 tbsp	80	0	0	0	0	4.5	0/0	0	90	0
I Can't Believe It's Not Butter, Easy Squeeze	1 tbsp	80	0	0	0	0	8	1.5/0	0	95	0
I Can't Believe It's Not Butter Fat-Free Spread	1 tbsp	5	0	0	0	0	0	0/0	0	90	0
I Can't Believe It's Not Butter Light Spread	1 tbsp	50	0	0	0	0	5	1/0	0	90	0
I Can't Believe It's Not Butter Sweet Cream & Calcium Spread	1 tbsp	50	0	0	0	0	6	1/0	0	85	0
Olivio Premium Spread with Olive Oil	1 tbsp	80	0	0	0	0	8	1/0	0	95	0
Parkay Light Spread	1 tbsp	50	0	0	0	0	5	1/0	0	130	0
Parkay Original Spread	1 tbsp	80	0	0	0	0	7	1.5/0	0	100	0

Food	Serving	Cal	Prot (g)	Carb (g)	Fiber (g)	Sugars (g)	Total Fat (g)	Sat/Trans Fat (g)	Chol (g)	Sod (mg)	GI
Parkay Squeeze Spread	1 tbsp	70	0	0	0	0	8	1.5/0	0	110	0
Promise Buttery Light Spread	1 tbsp	50	0	0	0	0	5	1/0	0	85	0
Promise Fat-Free Spread	1 tbsp	5	0	0	0	0	0	0/0	0	90	0
Smart Balance Buttery Spread	1 tbsp	80	0	0	0	0	9	2.5/0	0	90	0
Smart Balance Light Spread	1 tbsp	50	0	0	0	0	5	1.5/0	0	85	0
Smart Beat Fat-Free Squeeze Margarine	1 tbsp	5	0	0	0	0	0	0/0	0	na	0
Smart Beat Trans Free Super Light Margarine	1 tbsp	20	0	0	0	0	2	0/0	0	105	0
Smart Beat Unsalted Light Margarine	1 tbsp	30	0	0	0	0	3	0/0	0	na	0
Shedd's Spread Chum Style Country Crock	1 tbsp	60	0	0	0	0	7	1.5/0	0	90	0
Shedd's Spread Country Crock Easy Squeeze	1 tbsp	60	0	0	0	0	7	1/0	0	85	0
Shedd's Spread Country Crock Plus Calcium and Vitamins	1 tbsp	50	0	0	0	0	5	1/0	0	110	0

145

Food	Serving	Cal	Prot (g)	Carb (g)	Fiber (g)	Sugars (g)	Total Fat (g)	Sat/Trans Fat (g)	Chol (g)	Sod (mg)	GI
Shedd's Spread Light Country Crock	1 tbsp	50	0	0	0	0	5	1/0	0	1	0
Take Control Spread	1 tbsp	80	0	0	0	0	8	1/0	t	85	0
Take Control Light Spread	1 tbsp	45	0	0	0	0	5	.5/0	t	85	0
Shortenings											
Shortening, multipurpose, soybean (hydrogenated) and palm (hydrogenated)	1 tbsp	113	0	0	0	0	13	4/na	0	0	0
Shortening, vegetable, household,	1 tbsp	113	0	0	0	0	13	3/na	0	0	0
Shortening, household, soybean (hydrogenated) and cottonseed (hydrogenated)	1 tbsp	113	0	0	0	0	13	3/2	0	1	0
0 Grams Trans Fat All-Vegetable (Crisco)	1 tbsp	106	0	0	0	0	12	3/0	0	0	0
Mayonnaise											
Mayonnaise, regular	1 tbsp	57	t	4	0	na	5	1/na	4	105	0
Mayonnaise, regular, soybean-base	1 tbsp	99	t	t	0	na	11	2/na	8	78	0

146

Food	Serving	Cal	Prot (g)	Carb (g)	Fiber (g)	Sugars (g)	Total Fat (g)	Sat/Trans Fat (g)	Chol (g)	Sod (mg)	GI
Mayonnaise, fat-free (Kraft)	2 tbsp	22	t	4	t	2	t	t/na	3	240	0
Mayonnaise, made w/ tofu	2 tbsp	96	2	2	0	0	10	0/na	0	232	0
Mayonnaise, imitation, milk cream	2 tbsp	30	0	4	0	na	2	0/na	12	152	0
Mayonnaise, imitation, soybean-base	2 tbsp	70	t	5	0	na	6	1/na	7	149	0
Mayonnaise, imitation, soybean-base, w/o cholesterol	1 tbsp	68	t	2	0	na	7	1/na	0	50	0
Mayonnaise, light (Kraft)	2 tbsp	100	t	3	0	1	10	2/na	11	239	0
Miracle Whip, light (Kraft)	2 tbsp	74	t	5	0	3	6	1/t	8	263	0
Miracle Whip Free, nonfat (Kraft)	2 tbsp	27	t	5	t	3	t	t/na	3	252	0
Oils											
Almond oil	1 tbsp	119	0	0	0	0	14	1/0	0	0	0
Apricot kernel oil	1 tbsp	119	0	0	0	0	14	1/0	0	0	0
Avocado oil	1 tbsp	124	0	0	0	0	14	2/0	na	0	0
Butter replacement, w/o fat, powder	1 tsp	6	0	1	0	0	0	0/0	0	20	0

Food	Serving	Cal	Prot (g)	Carb (g)	Fiber (g)	Sugars (g)	Total Fat (g)	Sat/Trans Fat (g)	Chol (g)	Sod (mg)	GI
Canola oil	1 tbsp	124	0	0	0	0	14	1/0	0	0	0
Coconut oil	1 tbsp	116	0	0	0	0	14	12/0	0	0	0
Corn oil, salad or cooking	1 tbsp	120	0	0	0	0	14	2/0	0	0	0
Flaxseed oil	1 tbsp	119	0	0	0	0	14	1/0	0	0	0
Grapeseed oil	1 tbsp	120	0	0	0	0	14	1/0	0	0	0
Hazelnut oil	1 tbsp	119	0	0	0	0	14	1/0	0	0	0
Olive oil, salad or cooking	1 tbsp	119	0	0	0	0	14	2/0	0	0	0
Peanut oil, salad or cooking	1 tbsp	119	0	0	0	0	14	3/0	0	0	0
Sesame oil, salad or cooking	1 tbsp	120	0	0	0	0	14	2/0	0	0	0
Safflower oil (70% linoleic), salad or cooking	1 tbsp	120	0	0	0	0	14	1/0	0	0	0
Safflower oil (over 70% safflower) salad or cooking	1 tbsp	120	0	0	0	0	14	1/0	0	0	0
Soybean oil, salad or cooking	1 tbsp	120	0	0	0	0	14	2/0	0	0	0
Sunflower oil (less than 60% linoleic)	1 tbsp	120	0	0	0	0	14	1/0	0	0	0

Food	Serving	Cal	Prot (g)	Carb (g)	Fiber (g)	Sugars (g)	Total Fat (g)	Sat/Trans Fat (g)	Chol (g)	Sod (mg)	GI
Sunflower oil (more than 60% linoleic)	1 tbsp	120	0	0	0	0	14	1/0	0	0	0
Sunflower oil (more than 70% oleic)	1 tbsp	124	0	0	0	0	14	1/0	0	0	0
Walnut oil	1 tbsp	120	0	0	0	0	14	1/0	0	0	0
Wheat germ oil	1 tbsp	120	0	0	0	0	14	2/0	0	0	0

Food	Serving	Cal	Prot (g)	Carb (g)	Fiber (g)	Sugars (g)	Total Fat (g)	Sat/Trans Fat (g)	Chol (mg)	Sod (mg)
FISH AND SHELLFISH										
Fish										
Anchovy, canned in oil, drained	1 can (2 oz)	95	13	0	0	na	4	1/0	38	1651
Bass, freshwater, mixed species, cooked	4 oz	165	27	0	0	0	5	1/0	99	102
Bass, striped, cooked	4 oz	141	26	0	0	0	3	1/0	117	100
Bluefish, cooked	4 oz	180	29	0	0	0	6	1/0	86	87
Burbot, cooked	4 oz	130	28	0	0	0	1	t/0	87	141
Butterfish, cooked	4 oz	212	25	0	0	0	12	na/na	94	129
Carp, cooked	4 oz	184	26	0	0	0	8	2/0	95	71
Catfish, breaded and fried	4 oz	260	20.5	9	1	na	15	4/na	92	317
Catfish, channel, farmed, cooked	4 oz	172	21	0	0	0	9	2/0	73	91
Catfish, channel, wild, cooked	4 oz	119	21	0	0	0	3	1/0	82	57
Caviar, black and red, granular	3 tbsp	121	12	2	0	0	9	2/0	282	720
Cod, Atlantic, canned	4 oz	119	26	0	0	0	1	t/0	62	247

Food	Serving	Cal	Prot (g)	Carb (g)	Fiber (g)	Sugars (g)	Total Fat (g)	Sat/Trans Fat (g)	Chol (mg)	Sod (mg)
Cod, Atlantic, cooked	4 oz	119	26	0	0	0	1	t/0	62	88
Cod, Pacific, cooked	4 oz	119	26	0	0	0	1	t/0	53	103
Dolphinfish, cooked	4 oz	124	27	0	0	0	1	t/0	107	128
Drum, freshwater, cooked	4 oz	173	26	0	0	0	7	2/0	93	109
Fish fillet, fried, generic	1 fillet	211	13	15.5	.5	na	11	3/na	31	484
Fish sticks, frozen, preheated	4 sticks	305	17.5	27	0	na	14	3.5/0	125	652
Flounder, cooked	4 oz	133	27	0	0	0	2	t/0	77	119
Grouper, mixed species, cooked	4 oz	134	28	0	0	0	1	t/0	53	60
Haddock, cooked	4 oz	127	27	0	0	0	1	t/0	84	99
Halibut, Atlantic and Pacific, cooked	4 oz	159	30	0	0	0	3	t/0	46	78
Halibut, Greenland, cooked	4 oz	271	21	0	0	0	20	4/0	67	117
Herring, Atlantic, cooked	4 oz	230	26	0	0	0	13	3/0	87	130
Herring, Atlantic, kippered, large (7" × 2¼" × ¼")	1 fillet	141	16	0	0	0	8	2/0	53	597

151

Food	Serving	Cal	Prot (g)	Carb (g)	Fiber (g)	Sugars (g)	Total Fat (g)	Sat/Trans Fat (g)	Chol (mg)	Sod (mg)
Herring, Atlantic, pickled, (1¾"×⅞"×½")	3 pieces	118	6	4	0	0	8	1/0	6	391
Herring, Pacific, cooked	4 oz	283	24	0	0	0	20	5/0	112	108
Mackerel, Atlantic, cooked	4 oz	297	27	0	0	0	20	5/0	85	94
Mackerel, Jack, canned, boneless	4 oz	177	26	0	0	0	7	2/0	90	430
Mackerel, King, cooked	4 oz	152	29	0	0	0	3	1/0	77	230
Mackerel, Pacific and Jack, mixed species, cooked, boneless	4 oz	228	29	0	0	0	11	3/0	68	125
Mackerel, Spanish, cooked	4 oz	179	27	0	0	0	7	2/0	83	75
Monkfish, cooked	4 oz	110	21	0	0	0	2	na/na	36	26
Mahi-mahi	1 fillet	173	38	0	0	0	1.5	t/0	149	180
Mullet, striped, cooked	4 oz	170	28	0	0	0	6	2/0	71	80
Ocean perch, Atlantic, cooked	4 oz	137	27	0	0	0	2	t/0	61	109
Orange roughy, cooked	4 oz	101	21	0	0	0	1	t/0	29	92
Perch, mixed species, cooked	4 oz	133	28	0	0	0	1	t/0	130	90
Pike, Northern, cooked	4 oz	128	28	0	0	0	1	t/0	57	56

152

Food	Serving	Cal	Prot (g)	Carb (g)	Fiber (g)	Sugars (g)	Total Fat (g)	Sat/Trans Fat (g)	Chol (mg)	Sod (mg)
Pike, Walleye, cooked	4 oz	135	28	0	0	0	2	t/0	125	74
Pollock, Atlantic, cooked	4 oz	134	28	0	0	0	1	t/0	103	125
Pollock, Walleye, cooked	4 oz	128	27	0	0	0	1	t/0	109	131
Pompano, Florida, cooked	4 oz	239	27	0	0	0	14	5/0	73	86
Rockfish, Pacific, mixed species, cooked	4 oz	137	27	0	0	0	2	1/0	50	87
Roe, mixed species, cooked	4 oz	231	32	2	0	0	9	2/0	543	133
Salmon, Atlantic, farmed, cooked	4 oz	233	25	0	0	0	14	3/0	71	69
Salmon, Atlantic, wild, cooked	4 oz	206	29	0	0	0	9	1/0	80	63
Salmon, Chinook, cooked	4 oz	262	29	0	0	0	15	4/0	96	68
Salmon, Chinook, smoked (lox), cooked	4 oz	133	21	0	0	0	5	1/0	25	2,267
Salmon, Chum, cooked	4 oz	175	29	0	0	0	5	1/0	108	73
Salmon, Chum, drained solids, with bone	4 oz	160	24	0	0	0	6	2/0	44	552
Salmon, Coho, farmed, cooked	4 oz	202	28	0	0	0	9	2/0	71	59

153

Food	Serving	Cal	Prot (g)	Carb (g)	Fiber (g)	Sugars (g)	Total Fat (g)	Sat/Trans Fat (g)	Chol (mg)	Sod (mg)
Salmon, Coho, wild, cooked	4 oz	158	27	0	0	0	5	1/0	62	66
Salmon, pink, canned, solids with bone and liquid	4 oz	158	22	0	0	0	7	2/0	62	628
Salmon, pink, cooked	4 oz	169	29	0	0	0	5	1/0	76	97
Salmon, Sockeye, canned, drained solids with bone	4 oz	173	23	0	0	0	8	2/0	50	610
Salmon, Sockeye, cooked	4 oz	245	31	0	0	0	12	2/0	99	75
Salmon, smoked (lox)	4 oz	133	21	0	0	0	5	1/0	26	2,267
Sardines, canned in oil, drained	4 oz	236	28	0	0	0	13	2/0	161	573
Sardines, Pacific, canned in tomato sauce, drained solids w/bone	3 pieces	203	19	0	0	0	14	4/0	70	472
Sea bass, mixed species, cooked	4 oz	141	27	0	0	0	3	1/0	60	99
Sea trout, mixed species, cooked	4 oz	151	24	0	0	0	5	1/0	120	84
Shad, American, cooked	4 oz	286	26	0	0	0	20	na/na	109	74
Shark	4 oz	148	24	0	0	0	5	1/0	58	90
Shark, breaded and fried	4 oz	258	21	7	0	na	16	4/0	67	138

154

Food	Serving	Cal	Prot (g)	Carb (g)	Fiber (g)	Sugars (g)	Total Fat (g)	Sat/Trans Fat (g)	Chol (mg)	Sod (mg)
Smelt, Rainbow, cooked	4 oz	141	26	0	0	0	4	1/0	102	87
Snapper, mixed species, cooked	4 oz	145	30	0	0	0	2	t/0	53	65
Spot, cooked	4 oz	179	27	0	0	0	7	2/0	87	42
Sturgeon, mixed species, cooked, boneless	4 oz	153	23	0	0	0	6	1/0	87	78
Sunfish, pumpkin seed, cooked	4 oz	129	28	0	0	0	1	t/0	97	117
Surimi	4 oz	112	17	8	0	0	1	t/0	34	162
Swordfish, cooked	4 oz	176	29	0	0	0	5	2/0	57	130
Tilefish, cooked	4 oz	167	28	0	0	0	5	1/0	73	67
Trout, mixed species, cooked	4 oz	215	30	0	0	0	10	2/0	84	76
Trout, Rainbow, farmed, cooked	4 oz	192	28	0	0	0	8	2/0	77	48
Trout, Rainbow, wild, cooked	4 oz	170	26	0	0	0	7	2/0	78	63
Tuna, bluefin, fresh, cooked	4 oz	209	34	0	0	0	7	2/0	56	57
Tuna, light, canned in oil, drained	4 oz	225	33	0	0	0	9	2/0	20	401
Tuna, light, canned in water, drained solids	4 oz	132	29	0	0	0	1	t/0	34	383

155

Food	Serving	Cal	Prot (g)	Carb (g)	Fiber (g)	Sugars (g)	Total Fat (g)	Sat/Trans Fat (g)	Chol (mg)	Sod (mg)
Tuna, white, canned in oil, drained	4 oz	211	30	0	0	0	9	2/0	35	449
Tuna, white, canned in water, drained solids	4 oz	145	27	0	0	0	3	1/0	48	427
Tuna, yellowfish, fresh, cooked	4 oz	158	34	0	0	0	1	t/0	66	53
Turbot, European, cooked	4 oz	138	23	0	0	0	4	na/na	70	218
Whitefish, mixed species, cooked	4 oz	195	28	0	0	0	9	1/0	87	74
Whiting, mixed species, cooked	4 oz	131	27	0	0	0	2	t/0	95	150
Yellowtail, mixed species, cooked	4 oz	212	34	0	0	0	8	na/na	80	57
Shellfish										
Clams, breaded and fried	4 oz	229	16	12	na	na	13	3/0	69	413
Clams, mixed species, canned, drained solids	4 oz	168	29	6	0	0	2	t/0	76	127
Clams, mixed species, cooked	4 oz	168	29	6	0	0	2	t/0	76	127
Crab, Alaska King, cooked	4 oz	110	22	0	0	0	2	t/0	60	1,215
Crab, Alaska King, imitation, made from surimi	4 oz	116	14	12	0	0	1	t/0	23	953

Food	Serving	Cal	Prot (g)	Carb (g)	Fiber (g)	Sugars (g)	Total Fat (g)	Sat/Trans Fat (g)	Chol (mg)	Sod (mg)
Crab, Blue, cooked	4 oz	116	23	0	0	0	2	t/0	113	367
Crab, Dungeness, cooked	4 oz	125	25	1	0	0	1	t/0	86	428
Crab, Queen, cooked	4 oz	130	27	0	0	0	2	t/0t	80	783
Crab cakes, fried	2 cakes	186	24	.5	0	na	9	2/0	180	396
Lobster, Northern, cooked	4 oz	111	23	1	0	0	1	t/0	82	431
Lobster, spiny, mixed species, cooked	4 oz	162	30	4	0	0	2	t/0	102	257
Oysters, breaded and fried	4 oz	223	10	13	na	na	14	4/0	92	473
Oysters, Eastern, canned, drained	4 oz	63	7	4	0	0	2	1/0	51	103
Oysters, Eastern, farmed, cooked, dry heat	4 oz	90	8	8	0	0	2	1/0	43	185
Oysters, Eastern, wild, cooked, dry heat	4 oz	82	9	5	0	0	2	1/0	56	277
Oysters, Eastern, wild, cooked, moist heat	4 oz	155	16	9	0	0	6	2/0	119	478
Oysters, Pacific, cooked, moist heat	4 oz	185	21	11	0	0	5	1/0	113	240

Food	Serving	Cal	Prot (g)	Carb (g)	Fiber (g)	Sugars (g)	Total Fat (g)	Sat/Trans Fat (g)	Chol (mg)	Sod (mg)
Scallops, breaded and fried	4 oz	241	20	11	na	na	12	3/0	68	520
Scallops, mixed species, imitation, made from surimi	4 oz	112	14	12	0	0	t	t/0	25	901
Shrimp, breaded and fried	4 oz	274	24	13	.5	na	14	2/0	201	390
Shrimp, mixed species, canned	1 oz	34	7	0	0	0	1	t/0	49	48
Shrimp, mixed species, cooked, moist heat	4 oz	112	24	0	0	0	1	t/0	221	254
Shrimp, mixed species, imitation, made from surimi	4 oz	114	14	10	0	0	2	t/0	41	799
Squid, fried (calamari)	4 oz	198	20	9	0	na	8.5	2/0	295	347

158

Food	Serving	Cal	Prot (g)	Carb (g)	Fiber (g)	Sugars (g)	Total Fat (g)	Sat/Trans Fat (g)	Chol (g)	Sod (mg)	GI
FRUITS											
Acerola (West Indian cherry), raw	1 cup	31	t	8	1	na	t	t/0	0	7	20
Apple, dehydrated, sulfured, uncooked	½ cup	104	t	28	4	24	t	t/0	0	37	29
Apple, dried, sulfured, uncooked	5 rings	78	t	21	3	28	t	t/0	0	28	29
Apple, raw (2¾" diameter), with skin	1 fruit	81	t	21	4	14	t	t/0	0	0	38
Apple, raw (2¾" diameter), without skin	1 fruit	73	t	19	2	13	t	t/0	0	0	38
Apple, raw, with skin, sliced	1 cup	65	t	17	3	na	t	t/0	0	0	38
Apple, raw, without skin, sliced	1 cup	63	t	16	2	na	t	t/0	0	0	38
Applesauce, canned, sweetened, w/ salt	½ cup	97	t	25	1.5	na	t	t/0	0	36	na
Applesauce, canned, sweetened, w/o salt	½ cup	97	t	25	1.5	21	t	t/0	0	4	na
Applesauce, unsweetened	½ cup	52	t	14	1.5	12	t	t/0	0	2	35

159

Food	Serving	Cal	Prot (g)	Carb (g)	Fiber (g)	Sugars (g)	Total Fat (g)	Sat/Trans Fat (g)	Chol (g)	Sod (mg)	GI
Apricots, canned, extra heavy syrup, w/o skin, solids and liquids	1/2 cup, whole, w/o pits	118	1	31	2	na	t	t/0	0	16	na
Apricots, canned, heavy syrup, w/o skin, solids and liquids	1/2 cup, whole, w/o pits	107	1	28	2	na	t	t/0	0	14	na
Apricots, canned, light syrup, w/ skin, solids and liquids	1/2 cup, halves	80	1	21	2	18	t	t/0	0	5	64
Apricots, canned, water pack, without skin	1/2 cup	25	1	6	1	na	t	t/0	0	13	na
Apricots, canned, water pack, with skin	1/2 cup	33	1	8	2	6	t	t/0	0	3	na
Apricots, dried, sulfured, uncooked	10 halves	84	1	22	2.5	19	t	t/0	0	4	31
Apricots, raw	2	140	1	8	2	3	t	t/0	0	0	57
Apricots, raw, sliced	1 cup	79	2	18	4	na	1	t/0	0	2	57
Avocado, raw, all varieties	1/4 fruit	81	1	4	2.5	t	8	1/0	0	5	10

Food	Serving	Cal	Prot (g)	Carb (g)	Fiber (g)	Sugars (g)	Total Fat (g)	Sat/Trans Fat (g)	Chol (g)	Sod (mg)	GI
Avocado, raw, without skin and seeds, California	¼ fruit	77	1	3	2	t	8	1/0	0	5	10
Avocado, raw, without skin and seeds, Florida	¼ fruit	85	1	7	4	t	7	1/0	0	4	10
Banana (7" to 7⅞" long), raw	1 fruit	109	1	28	3	14	1	t/0	0	1	46
Blackberries, frozen, unsweetened, unthawed	1 cup	97	2	24	7.5	16	1	t/0	0	2	25
Blackberries, raw	1 cup	75	1	18	8	7	1	t/0	0	0	25
Blueberries, frozen, sweetened	1 cup, thawed	186	1	50	5	45	0/0	0/0	0	2	na
Blueberries, frozen, unsweetened, unthawed	1 cup	79	1	19	4.2	13	1	t/0	0	2	25
Blueberries, raw	1 cup	81	1	20	4	15	t	t/0	0	9	24
Cherries, sour, red, canned, in heavy syrup, solids and liquids	½ cup	117	1	30	1	29	0/0	0/0	0	9	na
Cherries, sour, red, canned, water pack	1 cup	88	2	22	3	19	t	t/0	0	17	25

Food	Serving	Cal	Prot (g)	Carb (g)	Fiber (g)	Sugars (g)	Total Fat (g)	Sat/Trans Fat (g)	Chol (g)	Sod (mg)	GI
Cherries, sour, red, frozen, unsweetened, unthawed	1 cup	71	1	17	2.5	14	1	t/0	0	2	25
Cherries, sour, red, raw, without pits	1 cup	78	2	19	2.5	13	t	t/0	0	5	22
Cherries, sour, red, raw, with pits	1 cup	52	1	13	1.5	9	t	t/0	0	3	22
Cherries, sweet, canned, juice pack, pitted	1 cup	135	2	35	4	31	t	t/0	0	8	25
Cherries, sweet, canned, water pack, pitted	1 cup	114	2	29	4	19	t	t/0	0	2	25
Cherries, sweet, raw, without pits	1 cup	104	2	24	3	19	1	t/0	0	0	25
Cherries, sweet, raw, with pits	1 cup	84	1	19	3	15	1	t/0	0	0	25
Cherry pie filling, low calorie	1 cup	121	2	27	3	24	t	0/0	0	32	na
Cranberries, dried, sweetened	1 cup	123	t	33	2	26	.5	0/0	0	1	na
Cranberries, raw, chopped	1 cup	54	0	14	4.6	4	t	t/0	0	1	45
Cranberries, raw, whole	1 cup	47	0	12	4	4	t	t/0	0	1	45
Cranberry sauce, canned, sweetened	½ cup	209	t	54	1	52	t	t/0	0	40	na
Currants, black, raw	1 cup	71	2	18	na	na	t	t/0	0	2	15

162

Food	Serving	Cal	Prot (g)	Carb (g)	Fiber (g)	Sugars (g)	Total Fat (g)	Sat/Trans Fat (g)	Chol (g)	Sod (mg)	GI
Currants, red and white, raw	1 cup	63	2	15	5	8	t	t/0	0	1	15
Dates, domestic, natural and dry	5 dates	114	1	31	3	80	1	t/0	0	1	100
Figs, canned, water pack	½ cup	66	0	17	3	15	t	t/0	0	1	61
Figs, dried, stewed	½ cup	140	2	36	7	30	t	t/0	0	6	na
Figs, dried, uncooked	2 figs	97	1	25	5	8	t	t/0	0	4	61
Figs, raw, large (2½" dia.)	2 figs	95	1	25	4	21	t	t/0	0	1	61
Fruit cocktail, canned, extra heavy syrup, solids and liquids	½ cup	114	1	30	1	na	t	t/0	0	8	na
Fruit cocktail, canned, heavy syrup, solids and liquids	½ cup	91	1	23	1	22	t	t/0	0	7	na
Fruit cocktail, canned, light syrup, solids and liquids	½ cup	69	t	18	1	16	t	t/0	0	7	55
Fruit cocktail, canned, juice pack	½ cup	55	1	14	1	13	1	t/0	0	5	55
Fruit cocktail, canned, water pack	½ cup	38	1	10	1	9	1	t/0	0	5	55
Fruit salad, canned, extra heavy syrup, solids and liquids	½ cup	114	t	30	1	na	t	t/0	0	6	na

163

Food	Serving	Cal	Prot (g)	Carb (g)	Fiber (g)	Sugars (g)	Total Fat (g)	Sat/Trans Fat (g)	Chol (g)	Sod (mg)	GI
Fruit salad, canned, heavy syrup, solids and liquids	½ cup	111	1	29	2	23	t	t/0	0	3	na
Fruit salad, canned, light syrup, solids and liquids	½ cup	73	t	19	1	na	t	t/0	0	8	na
Grapefruit, Pink, raw, red, and white, (4"diameter)	½ fruit	41	1	10	1.4	12	t	t/0	0	0	25
Grapefruit sections, canned, in light syrup, solids and liquids	½ cup	76	1	20	1	19	0/0	0/0	0	2	25
Grapefruit, canned sections, juice pack	½ cup	46	1	11	0.5	11	t	t/0	0	9	25
Grapefruit, canned sections, water pack	½ cup	44	1	11	0.5	4.5	t	t/0	0	2	25
Grapes, American, slip skin, raw	1 cup	62	1	16	1	15	t	t/0	0	2	43
Grapes, European, red or green, Thompson seedless, raw	1 cup	114	1	28	1.5	23	1	t/0	0	3	43
Grapes, Thompson seedless, canned, in heavy syrup, solids and liquids	½ cup	93	1	25	.5	24	t	t/0	0	6	43

164

Food	Serving	Cal	Prot (g)	Carb (g)	Fiber (g)	Sugars (g)	Total Fat (g)	Sat/Trans Fat (g)	Chol (g)	Sod (mg)	GI
Grapes, canned, Thompson, seedless, water pack	½ cup	49	1	13	1	12	t	t/0	0	7	43
Guava, common, raw, without refuse	1 fruit	46	1	11	5	5	1	t/0	0	3	56
Kiwi fruit, fresh, raw, without skin, large	1 fruit	56	1	14	3	8	t	t/0	0	5	53
Lemon, raw, without peel (2⅜" dia.)	1 fruit	24	1	8	2.5	2	t	t/0	0	2	na
Lime, raw (2" dia.)	1 fruit	20	0	7	2	1	t	t/0	0	1	na
Mango, raw, sliced	1 cup	107	1	28	3	24	t	t/0	0	3	51
Melon balls, frozen, unthawed	1 cup	57	1	14	1	na	t	t/0	0	54	60
Melon, cantaloupe, raw, wedge (⅛ of large melon)	1 wedge	36	1	9	1	8	t	t/0	0	9	60
Melon, casaba, raw, wedge (⅛ of melon)	1 wedge	53	2	13	2	9	t	t/0	0	25	60
Melon, honeydew, raw, wedge (⅛ of 6"–7" dia. melon)	1 wedge	56	1	15	1	12	t	t/0	0	16	60

Food	Serving	Cal	Prot (g)	Carb (g)	Fiber (g)	Sugars (g)	Total Fat (g)	Sat/Trans Fat (g)	Chol (g)	Sod (mg)	GI
Nectarine, raw (2½" dia.)	1 fruit	67	1	16	2	11	1	t/0	0	0	35
Orange, raw, California, navel (2⅞" dia.)	1 fruit	64	1	16	3.5	12	t	t/0	0	1	42
Orange, raw, California, valencia (2⅝" dia.)	1 fruit	59	1	14	3	na	t	t/0	0	0	42
Orange, raw, Florida (2⅝" dia.)	1 fruit	65	1	16	3.5	13	t	t/0	0	0	42
Papaya, raw, cubes	1 cup	55	1	14	2.5	8	t	t/0	0	4	55
Papaya, raw, small (4½" lg × 2¾" dia.)	1 fruit	59	1	15	3	9	t	t/0	0	5	55
Peaches, canned, extra heavy syrup, solids and liquids	½ cup, halves or slices	126	1	34	1	na	t	t/0	0	10	58
Peaches, canned, heavy syrup, solids and liquids	½ cup	97	1	26	2	24	t	t/0	0	8	58
Peaches, canned, light syrup, solids and liquids	½ cup, halves or slices	68	1	18	2	16	t	t/0	0	6	52

Food	Serving	Cal	Prot (g)	Carb (g)	Fiber (g)	Sugars (g)	Total Fat (g)	Sat/Trans Fat (g)	Chol (g)	Sod (mg)	GI
Peaches, canned, extra light syrup, solids and liquids	½ cup, halves or slices	52	t	14	1	na	t	t/0	0	6	52
Peaches, spiced, canned, extra heavy syrup, solids and liquids	½ cup, whole	91	1	24	2	na	t	t/0	0	5	58
Peaches, canned, juice pack, halves or slices	½ cup	55	1	14	1.5	13	t	t/0	0	5	45
Peaches, canned, water pack, halves or slices	½ cup	29	1	7	1.5	6	t	t/0	0	4	na
Peaches, dried, sulfured, stewed, without added sugar	½ cup	99	1	25	3.5	na	t	t/0	0	3	na
Peaches, dried, sulfured, uncooked, halves	3	93	1	24	3	na	t	t/0	0	3	na
Peaches, raw, large (2¾" dia.)	1 fruit	68	1	17	3	15	t	t/0	0	0	42
Peaches, raw, slices	1 cup	73	1	19	3	na	t	t/0	0	0	42
Pears, Asian, raw (2¼" long×2½" dia.)	1 fruit	51	1	13	4	17	t	t/0	0	0	38

Food	Serving	Cal	Prot (g)	Carb (g)	Fiber (g)	Sugars (g)	Total Fat (g)	Sat/Trans Fat (g)	Chol (g)	Sod (mg)	GI
Pears, canned, extra heavy syrup, solids and liquids	½ cup, halves	129	t	34	2	na	t	t/0	0	7	na
Pears, canned, heavy syrup, solids and liquids	½ cup	98	t	26	2	20	t	t/0	0	7	na
Pears, canned, light syrup, solids and liquids	½ cup, halves	72	t	19	2	15	t	t/0	0	6	na
Pears, canned, extra light syrup, solids and liquids	½ cup, halves	58	t	15	2	na	t	t/0	0	2	na
Pears, canned, juice pack, halves	½ cup	62	0	16	2	12	t	t/0	0	0	43
Pears, canned, water pack, halves	½ cup	35	0	10	2	7	t	t/0	0	2	na
Pear, raw, medium (approx. 2½" per pound)	1 fruit	98	1	25	4	17	1	t/0	0	0	33
Persimmons, Japanese, raw (2½" dia.)	1 fruit	118	1	31	6	21	t	t/0	0	2	50
Persimmons, native, raw, without refuse	1 fruit	32	0	8	na	na	t	t/0	0	0	50

Food	Serving	Cal	Prot (g)	Carb (g)	Fiber (g)	Sugars (g)	Total Fat (g)	Sat/Trans Fat (g)	Chol (g)	Sod (mg)	GI
Pineapple, canned, extra heavy syrup, solids and liquids	½ cup, crushed, sliced or chunks	108	t	28	1	na	t	t/0	0	1	na
Pineapple, canned, heavy syrup, solids and liquids	½ cup, crushed, sliced or chunks	99	t	26	1	22	t	t/0	0	1	na
Pineapple, canned, light syrup, solids and liquids	½ cup, crushed, sliced or chunks	66	t	17	1	16	t	t/0	0	1	na
Pineapple, canned, juice pack, chunks, crushed, slices	½ cup	75	0	20	1	na	t	t/0	0	1	na
Pineapple, canned, water pack, chunks, crushed, slices	½ cup	39	0	10	1	9	t	t/0	0	1	na
Pineapple, frozen, chunks, sweetened	½ cup, chunks	104	t	27	1	26	t	t/0	0	2	na
Pineapple, raw, diced	1 cup	76	1	19	2	14	t	t/0	0	2	59
Plantains, cooked, slices	½ cup	89	1	24	2	22	t	t/0	0	4	45

169

Food	Serving	Cal	Prot (g)	Carb (g)	Fiber (g)	Sugars (g)	Total Fat (g)	Sat/Trans Fat (g)	Chol (g)	Sod (mg)	GI
Plantains, raw, medium	½ fruit	109	1	29	2	27	t	t/0	0	4	45
Plums, canned, purple, juice pack, pitted	½ cup	73	0	19	1	na	t	t/0	0	1	na
Plums, canned, purple, extra heavy syrup, solids and liquids	½ cup, pitted	132	t	34	1	na	t	t/0	0	25	na
Plums, canned, purple, heavy syrup, solids and liquids	½ cup, pitted	115	t	30	1	28	t	t/0	0	25	na
Plums, canned, purple, light syrup, solids and liquids	½ cup, pitted	79	t	21	1	19	t	t/0	0	25	na
Plums, canned, purple, water pack, pitted	½ cup	51	0	14	1	12	t	t/0	0	1	na
Plum, raw (2⅛"dia.)	1 fruit	36	0	9	1	7	t	t/0	0	0	39
Pomegranate, raw (3⅜"dia.)	1 fruit	105	1	26	1	26	t	t/0	0	5	35
Prunes, canned, heavy syrup, solids and liquids	½ cup	123	1	33	4	na	t	t/0	0	4	na
Prunes, dried, stewed, w/added sugar	½ cup, pitted	154	1	41	5	na	t	t/0	0	2	na

170

Food	Serving	Cal	Prot (g)	Carb (g)	Fiber (g)	Sugars (g)	Total Fat (g)	Sat/Trans Fat (g)	Chol (g)	Sod (mg)	GI
Prunes, dried, stewed, without added sugar, pitted	½ cup	133	1	35	8	12	1	t/0	0	2	29
Prunes, dried, uncooked	5 fruit	100	1	26	3	na	t	t/0	0	2	29
Raisins, golden seedless, not packed	¼ cup	109	1	29	1.5	21	t	t/0	0	4	64
Raisins, seedless, not packed	¼ cup	109	1	29	1.5	21	t	t/0	0	4	64
Raisins, seedless, 5 oz, miniature box	1 box	42	0	11	1	8	t	t/0	0	2	64
Raspberries, raw	1 cup	60	1	14	8.4	5	1	t/0	0	0	25
Rhubarb, frozen, cooked, w/sugar	½ cup	139	t	37	2	35	t	t/0	0	0	na
Rhubarb, frozen, uncooked, diced	1 cup	29	1	7	2.5	1.5	t	t/0	0	3	15
Rhubarb, raw, diced	1 cup	26	1	6	2	1	t	t/0	0	5	15
Strawberries, frozen, sweetened, whole	1 cup	199	1	54	5	48	0/0	0/0	0	0	40
Strawberries, frozen, unsweetened, thawed	1 cup	77	1	20	5	10	t	t/0	0	4	25
Strawberries, raw, sliced	1 cup	50	1	12	4	7	1	t/0	0	2	25

171

Food	Serving	Cal	Prot (g)	Carb (g)	Fiber (g)	Sugars (g)	Total Fat (g)	Sat/Trans Fat (g)	Chol (g)	Sod (mg)	GI
Tangerine (mandarin), canned, juice pack	½ cup	46	1	12	1	11	t	t/0	0	6	na
Tangerine (mandarin), raw, large (2½" dia.)	1 fruit	43	1	11	2	13	t	t/0	0	1	30
Watermelon, raw, diced	1 cup	49	1	11	1	9	1	t/0	0	3	72
Watermelon, raw, wedge (1/16 of melon)	1 wedge	92	2	21	1.5	18	1	t/0	0	6	72
FRUIT JUICES, DRINKS, AND PUNCHES											
Acerola cherry juice	1 cup	56	1	12	1	na	1	t/0	0	7	na
Apple cider drink, low-calorie, w/ vitamin C, prepared w/water from powder	1 cup (8 fl oz)	2	0	1	0	0	0	0/0	0	34	na
Apple juice, canned or bottled	1 cup	117	t	29	t	27	t	t/0	0	7	39
Apple juice, from concentrate	1 cup	112	t	28	t	na	t	t/0	0	17	39
Apple raspberry cherry juice cocktail, ready-to-drink	1 cup (8 fl oz)	130	t	33	0	10	0/0	0/0	0	13	na

172

Food	Serving	Cal	Prot (g)	Carb (g)	Fiber (g)	Sugars (g)	Total Fat (g)	Sat/Trans Fat (g)	Chol (g)	Sod (mg)	GI
Apricot nectar, canned	1 cup (8 fl oz)	141	1	36	1.5	na	t/t	t/t	0	8	na
Cranberry-apple juice drink, bottled	1 cup (8 fl oz)	164	t	42	t	36	0/0	0/0	0	5	na
Cranberry-apricot juice drink, bottled	1 cup (8 fl oz)	157	t	40	t	na	0/0	0/0	0	5	na
Cranberry-grape juice drink, bottled	1 cup (8 fl oz)	137	t	34	t	na	t/t	t/t	0	7	na
Cranberry juice cocktail, bottled	1 cup (8 fl oz)	144	0	36	t	30	t/t	t/t	0	5	52
Cranberry juice, cocktail, low-calorie	1 cup	45	0	11	0	11	0	0/0	0	7	na
Cranberry juice cocktail, frozen concentrate, prepared w/water	1 cup (8 fl oz)	138	0	35	t	na	0/0	0/0	0	8	52
Fruit punch drink, canned	1 cup (8 fl oz)	117	0	30	t	28	0/0	0/0	0	55	na
Fruit punch drink, frozen concentrate, prepared w/water	1 cup (8 fl oz)	114	0	29	t	na	0/0	0/0	0	10	na
Fruit punch, ready-to-drink	1 serving	99	0	26	0	25	0/0	0/0	0	21	na

173

Food	Serving	Cal	Prot (g)	Carb (g)	Fiber (g)	Sugars (g)	Total Fat (g)	Sat/Trans Fat (g)	Chol (g)	Sod (mg)	GI
Fruit punch-flavor drink, powder, w/o added sodium, prepared w/water	1 cup (8 fl oz)	97	0	25	0	24	0/0	0/0	0	10	na
Grape berry punch, ready-to-drink	1 serving	116	0	31	0	30	0/0	0/0	0	35	na
Grape juice drink, canned	1 cup (8 fl oz)	125	t	32	t	35	0/0	0/0	0	3	55
Grape juice, canned or bottled	1 cup	154	1	38	t	38	t	t/0	0	8	55
Grapefruit juice, canned	1 cup	94	1	22	t	22	t	t/0	0	2	48
Grapefruit juice, from concentrate	1 cup	101	1	24	t	24	t	t/0	0	2	48
Grapefruit juice, pink, fresh	1 cup	96	1	23	0	na	t	t/0	0	2	48
Grapefruit juice, white, fresh	1 cup	96	1	23	t	22	t	t/0	0	2	48
Lemon juice, bottled	1 tbsp	3	0	1	0	0	0	0/0	0	3	20
Lemon juice, raw	Yield from 1 lemon	12	0	4	0	1	0	0/0	0	0	20
Lemonade mix, with vitamin C	1 portion, 1/8 cap/ tub	64	t	18	t	15	t	t/t	na	13	54

174

Food	Serving	Cal	Prot (g)	Carb (g)	Fiber (g)	Sugars (g)	Total Fat (g)	Sat/Trans Fat (g)	Chol (g)	Sod (mg)	GI
Lemonade, pink, frozen concentrate, prepared w/water	1 cup	99	t	26	0	na	0	0/0	0	7	54
Lemonade, powder, prepared w/water	1 cup	103	0	27	0	27	0	0/0	0	13	54
Lemonade, white, frozen concentrate, prepared w/water	1 cup	99	t	34	t	33	0	0/0	0	7	54
Lemonade-flavor drink, powder, prepared w/water	1 cup	112	0	29	0	na	0	0/0	0	19	54
Lime juice, raw	Yield from 1 lime	10	0	3	0	1	0	0/0	0	0	na
Orange juice, California, from concentrate	1 cup	110	2	25	na	na	t	t/0	0	2	53
Orange juice, canned, unsweetened	1 cup	105	1	25	.5	21	t	t/0	0	5	53
Orange juice, from concentrate	1 cup	110	2	25	.5	na	t	t/0	0	2	53
Orange juice, fresh	1 cup	112	2	26	.5	21	t	t/0	0	2	53
Orange and apricot juice drink, canned	1 cup	128	1	32	t	30	t	t/0	0	5	na

175

Food	Serving	Cal	Prot (g)	Carb (g)	Fiber (g)	Sugars (g)	Total Fat (g)	Sat/Trans Fat (g)	Chol (g)	Sod (mg)	GI
Orange-grapefruit juice, canned	1 cup	106	1	25	t	25	t	t/0	0	7	na
Papaya nectar, canned	1 cup	143	t	36	1.5	35	t	t/0	0	13	na
Passion-fruit juice, purple, fresh	1 cup	126	1	34	.5	33	t	t/0	0	15	na
Passion-fruit juice, yellow, fresh	1 cup	148	2	36	.5	na	t	t/0	0	15	na
Peach nectar, canned	1 cup	134	1	35	1.5	na	t	t/0	0	17	na
Pear nectar, canned	1 cup	150	t	39	1.5	na	t	t/0	0	10	na
Pineapple juice, canned, unsweetened	1 cup	140	1	34	.5	25	t	t/0	0	3	46
Pineapple juice, from concentrate	1 cup	130	1	32	.5	31	t	t/0	0	3	46
Pineapple and grapefruit juice drink, canned	1 cup	118	1	29	t	29	t	t/0	0	35	na
Pineapple and orange juice drink, canned	1 cup	125	3	30	t	29	0	0/0	0	8	na
Prune juice, canned	½ cup	91	1	22	1	42	t	t/0	0	5	na
Tangerine juice, fresh	1 cup	106	1	25	.5	24	t	t/0	0	2	na
Tropical punch, ready-to-drink	1 serving	90	0	24	0	23	0	0/0	0	29	na
Tropical punch, powder, prepared w/water	1 serving	64	0	16	0	16	0	0/0	0	2	na

Food	Serving	Cal	Prot (g)	Carb (g)	Fiber (g)	Sugars (g)	Total Fat (g)	Sat/Trans Fat (g)	Chol (mg)	Sod (mg)
GAME MEATS										
Bison, chuck roast, lean only, braised	4 oz	218	38	0	0	0	6	3/0	125	64
Bison, ribeye, lean only	4 oz	131	25	0	0	0	3	1/0	70	54
Bison, lean only, roasted	4 oz	162	32	0	0	0	3	1/0	93	65
Bison, top round, lean only, broiled	4 oz	197	34	0	0	0	6	2/0	96	46
Bison, top sirloin, lean only, broiled	4 oz	193	32	0	0	0	6	3/0	97	60
Rabbit, domesticated, various cuts, roasted	4 oz	223	33	0	0	0	9	3/0	93	53
Rabbit, domesticated, various cuts, stewed	4 oz	233	34	0	0	0	10	3/0	97	42
Rabbit, wild, various cuts, stewed	4 oz	196	37	0	0	0	4	1/0	139	51
Venison, ground, pan-broiled	4 oz	211	30	0	0	0	9	4.50	111	88
Venison, loin, lean only, broiled	4 oz	170	34	0	0	0	3	1/0	89	64

Food	Serving	Cal	Prot (g)	Carb (g)	Fiber (g)	Sugars (g)	Total Fat (g)	Sat/Trans Fat (g)	Chol (mg)	Sod (mg)
Venison, roasted	4 oz	179	34	0	0	0	4	1/0	127	61
Venison, shoulder roast, lean only, braised	4 oz	216	41	0	0	0	4	2/0	128	59
Venison, tenderloin, lean only, broiled	4 oz	168	34	0	0	0	3	1/0	99	64
Venison, top round, lean only, broiled	4 oz	172	36	0	0	0	2	1/0	96	51
GOOSE, DUCK, AND SPECIALTY POULTRY										
Duck, meat and skin, roasted	4 oz	377	21	0	0	0	32	11/0	94	66
Duck, wild, breast, w/o skin, cooked	4 oz	140	22	0	0	0	5	5/0	88	64
Goose, domesticated, meat and skin, roasted	4 oz	342	28	0	0	0	25	8/0	102	78
Goose, w/o skin, roasted	4 oz	268	33	0	0	0	14	14/0	108	88
Liver, chicken, cooked	4 oz	176	28	0	0	0	6	6/0	716	56

Food	Serving	Cal	Prot (g)	Carb (g)	Fiber (g)	Sugars (g)	Total Fat (g)	Sat/Trans Fat (g)	Chol (mg)	Sod (mg)
Ostrich, cooked	4 oz	160	30	0	0	0	3	3/0	108	88
Pâté de foie gras (goose liver pâté), canned, smoked	1 tbsp	60	1	1	0	na	6	2/0	20	91
Pheasant, w/o skin, cooked	4 oz	152	27	0	0	0	4	4/0	76	40

Food	Serving	Cal	Prot (g)	Carb (g)	Fiber (g)	Sugars (g)	Total Fat (g)	Sat/Trans Fat (g)	Chol (g)	Sod (mg)	GI
GRAINS AND GRAIN CAKES											
Grains											
Amaranth, dry	1/4 cup	182	7	32	7	na	3	1/0	0	10	35
Barley, pearled, cooked	1/2 cup	97	2	22	3	t	t	t/0	0	2	25
Bulgur, cooked	1/2 cup	76	3	17	4	t	t	t/0	0	5	54
Couscous, cooked	1/2 cup	88	3	18	1	t	t	t/0	0	4	65
Millet, cooked	1/2 cup	104	3	21	1	t	t	t/0	0	2	71
Quinoa, cooked	1/2 cup	106	6	17	1.5	na	1.5	0/0	0	6	35
Rice, brown, long-grain, cooked	1/2 cup	108	3	22	2	t	1	t/0	0	5	55
Rice, brown, medium-grain, cooked	1/2 cup	109	2	23	2	t	1	t/0	0	1	55
Rice noodles, cooked	1/2 cup	96	1	22	1	na	t	t/0	0	17	na
White rice, w/pasta, cooked	1/2 cup	123	3	22	3	na	3	1/0	1	574	na
White rice, short-grained, cooked	1/2 cup	121	2	27	na	t	t	t/0	0	0	64
White rice, medium-grained, cooked	1/2 cup	121	2	27	t	t	t	t/0	0	0	64

Food	Serving	Cal	Prot (g)	Carb (g)	Fiber (g)	Sugars (g)	Total Fat (g)	Sat/Trans Fat (g)	Chol (g)	Sod (mg)	GI
White rice, long-grained, cooked	½ cup	103	2	22	t	t	t	t/0.	0	1	56
White rice, long-grained, instant, cooked	½ cup	81	2	18	.5	t	t	t/0	0	2	56
White rice, long-grained, par boiled, enriched, cooked	½ cup	100	2	22	t	t	t	t/0	0	3	68
Wild rice, cooked	½ cup	83	3	18	1.5	t	t	t/0	0	2	35
Grain Cakes											
Brown rice, buckwheat, w/salt	2 cakes	68	2	14	na	na	1	t	0	21	85
Brown rice, buckwheat, w/o salt	2 cakes	68	2	14	1	na	1	t	0	1	85
Brown rice, corn	2 cakes	69	2	15	.5	na	1	t	0	52	85
Brown rice, multigrain, w/salt	2 cakes	70	2	15	.5	na	1	t	0	45	85
Brown rice, multigrain, w/o salt	2 cakes	70	2	15	na	na	1	t	0	1	85
Brown rice, plain, w/salt	2 cakes	70	1	15	1	t	t	t	0	59	85
Brown rice, plain, w/o salt	2 cakes	70	1	15	1	t	t	t	0	5	85
Brown rice, rye	2 cakes	69	1	15	1	na	1	t	0	20	85

181

Food	Serving	Cal	Prot (g)	Carb (g)	Fiber (g)	Sugars (g)	Total Fat (g)	Sat/Trans Fat (g)	Chol (g)	Sod (mg)	GI
Brown rice, sesame seed, w/o salt	2 cakes	71	1	15	na	na	1	t	0	1	85
Corn cakes	2 cakes	70	1	15	t	na	t	t	0	88	na
Corn cakes, very low-sodium	2 cakes	70	1	15	na	na	t	t	0	5	na
Popcorn cakes	2 cakes	77	2	16	1	t	1	t	0	58	na
GRAVIES AND SAUCES											
Gravies											
Au jus, canned	2 tbsp	5	t	1	0	na	t	t/0	0	15	na
Beef, from jar	2 tbsp	13	1	2	na	t	t	t/0	2	189	na
Beef, canned	2 tbsp	15	1	1	t	t	1	t/0	1	163	na
Brown gravy, canned	2 tbsp	12	t	2	na	t	t	t/0	1	176	na
Chicken, canned	2 tbsp	24	1	2	t	t	2	t/0	1	172	na
Mushroom, canned	2 tbsp	15	t	2	t	na	1	t/0	0	170	na
Sausage gravy, ready-to-serve	2 tbsp	48	1	2	t	t	4	1/0	7	118	na
Turkey, canned	2 tbsp	15	1	2	t	t	1	t/0	1	172	na

Food	Serving	Cal	Prot (g)	Carb (g)	Fiber (g)	Sugars (g)	Total Fat (g)	Sat/Trans Fat (g)	Chol (g)	Sod (mg)	GI
Sauces											
Adobo fresco	1 tbsp	41	0	3	0	1	4/1	1/0	0	3,087	na
Barbecue sauce	2 tbsp	24	1	4	t	na	1/t	t/0	0	265	na
Barbecue sauce, hickory smoke	2 tbsp	39	t	9	t	7	t/t	t/0	0	418	na
Bearnaise, dehydrated, dry	1 packet	91	4	15	0	0	2/0	0/0	0	847	na
Cheese sauce, ready-to-serve	¼ cup	110	4	4	t	t	8/4	4/0	18	522	na
Golden cheese sauce, ready-to-serve	¼ cup	139	7	2	1	t	11/6	6/0	29	501	na
Creole sauce, ready-to-serve	¼ cup	25	1	4	1	3	1/t	t/0	0	339	na
Fish sauce, ready-to-serve	2 tbsp	13	2	1	0	na	0/0	0/0	0	2,779	na
Hoisin sauce, ready-to-serve	2 tbsp	70	1	14	1	na	1/t	t/0	1	517	na
Hollandaise, w/butterfat, dehydrated, prepared w/water	1 packet	188	4	44	1	3	16/9	9/0	41	1,232	na
Jalapeño cheese sauce, ready-to-serve	¼ cup	81	2	8	0	t	5/2	2/0	6	571	na

Food	Serving	Cal	Prot (g)	Carb (g)	Fiber (g)	Sugars (g)	Total Fat (g)	Sat/Trans Fat (g)	Chol (g)	Sod (mg)	GI
Lemon sauce, ready-to-serve	2 tbsp	43	t	10	0	8	t/t	t/0	0	3	na
Mild nacho cheese sauce, ready-to-serve	1/4 cup	119	5	3	.5	0	10/4	4/na	20	492	na
Nacho cheese sauce, ready-to-serve	1/4 cup	128	5	4	t	t	10/6	6/na	29	580	na
Nacho cheese sauce, w/jalapeño peppers, mild, ready-to-serve	1/4 cup	122	1	7	t	2	10/3	3/na	4	551	na
Plum sauce, ready-to-serve	2 tbsp	70	t	16	t	na	t/t	t/0	0	204	na
Sharp cheddar cheese sauce, ready-to-serve	1/4 cup	133	5	2	1	t	12/5	5/na	23	473	na
Stir fry sauce, ready-to-serve	1 tbsp	16	t	2	0	1	1/t	t/0	0	233	na
Sweet and sour sauce, dry	1 packet	222	1	55	1	na	0/0	0/0	0	587	na
Sweet and sour glaze, ready-to-serve	2 tbsp	51	t	12	0	8	t/t	t/0	0	229	na
Sweet and sour sauce, ready-to-serve	2 tbsp	40	t	8	t	7	1/t	t/0	0	116	na

184

Food	Serving	Cal	Prot (g)	Carb (g)	Fiber (g)	Sugars (g)	Total Fat (g)	Sat/Trans Fat (g)	Chol (g)	Sod (mg)	GI
Tartar sauce	1 tbsp	74	t	2	0	na	8/1	1/0	6	103	na
White sauce, homemade, thin	¼ cup	66	2	5	t	na	4/1	1/0	5	205	na
White sauce, homemade, medium	¼ cup	92	2	6	t	na	7/2	2/0	4	221	na
White sauce, homemade, thick	¼ cup	116	2	7	t	na	92	2/0	4	233	na

Food	Serving	Cal	Prot (g)	Carb (g)	Fiber (g)	Sugars (g)	Total Fat (g)	Sat/Trans Fat (mg)	Chol (g)	Sod (mg)
HOT DOGS										
Cheesefurter, cheese smoke	1 link	141	6	1	0	1	12	5/na	29	465
Hot dog, beef	1 hot dog	149	5	2	0	1.5	13	5/na	24	513
Hot dog, beef, fat-free (Oscar Mayer)	1 hot dog	39	7	2.5	0	2	t	0/0	15	464
Hot dog, beef, light (Oscar Mayer)	1 hot dog	111	6	2	0	1	8.5	4/na	28	615
Hot dog, beef, low-fat	1 hot dog	133	7	1	0	0	11	5/na	23	593
Hot dog, beef and pork	1 hot dog	135	5	1	0	0	12.5	5/na	23	504
Hot dog, beef and pork, low-fat	1 hot dog	88	6	2.5	0	0	6	2/na	25	716
Hot dog, chicken	1 hot dog	116	6	3	0	0	9	2.5/na	45	617
Hot dog, low-sodium	1 hot dog	180	7	1	0	0	167	7/na	35	177

Food	Serving	Cal	Prot (g)	Carb (g)	Fiber (g)	Sugars (g)	Total Fat (g)	Sat/Trans Fat (mg)	Chol (g)	Sod (mg)
Hot dog, meatless	1 hot dog	163	14	5	3	0	10	1/na	0	330
Hot dog, pork	1 hot dog	204	10	t	t	0	18	7	50	620
Hot dog, fat-free (Oscar Mayer)	1 serving	37	6	2	0	1	t	t	15	487
Hot dog, turkey	1 hot dog	134	7.5	3	0	1	10	3/na	58	651
Hot dog, light pork, turkey, beef	1 serving	111	7	2	0	1	8.5	4/na	35	591

ICE CREAM AND FROZEN NOVELTIES

Food	Serving	Cal	Prot (g)	Carb (g)	Fiber (g)	Sugars (g)	Total Fat (g)	Sat/Trans Fat (g)	Chol (g)	Sod (mg)	GI
Butter pecan, no sugar added (Breyers)	½ cup	122	3	14.5	.6	6	7	3/na	12	112	na
Chocolate caramel, no sugar added (Breyers)	½ cup	107	2.5	18	.7	4	4	2.5/na	11	55	39
Chocolate ice cream (Atkins)	½ cup	140	2	13	5	1	12	7/na	40	20	na
Chocolate, light, no sugar added	½ cup	109	2.5	18	t	4	4	2.5/0	12	54	39
Creamsicle, sugar-free	1 pop	20	.5	5	3	t	1	.5/na	0	2.5	na
Fruit bar	1 bar	44	0	11	0	8	0	0/0	0	5	na
Fudge and Cream Pops (Atkins)	1 bar	70	2	7	2	1	6	3.5/na	20	10	na
Fudge Bars (Healthy Choice)	1 bar	80	3	13	0	2	1	.5/0	5	60	na
Klondike Slim-A-Bear Fudge Bar, sugar-free, 98% fat-free	1 bar (3.5 fl oz)	92	3	22	4	5	1	.7/0	5	89	na

Food	Serving	Cal	Prot (g)	Carb (g)	Fiber (g)	Sugars (g)	Total Fat (g)	Sat/Trans Fat (g)	Chol (g)	Sod (mg)	GI
Popsicles, sugar-free, all fruit flavors	1 pop (1.75 fl oz)	12	0	3	0	1	0	0/0	0	6	na
Praline and Caramel Ice Cream (Healthy Choice)	½ cup	121	3	23	1	19	2	1/t	5	63	na
Sherbet, orange	½ cup	122	1	26	0	19	1.5	1/na	5	35	na
Sherbet, rainbow	½ cup	122	1	26	0	20	1.5	1/na	5	35	na
Sorbet	½ cup	120	0	30	0	28	0	0/0	0	15	62
Vanilla chocolate strawberry, no sugar added (Breyers)	½ cup	97	2.5	15	.5	4	4	2.5/na	12	46	na
Vanilla, French, no sugar added (Breyers)	½ cup	105	3	14	t	5	5	3/na	36	59	na
Vanilla fudge twirl, no sugar added (Breyers)	½ cup	110	2.5	18.5	t	4	4	2.5/na	12	52	na
Vanilla Ice Cream (Atkins)	½ cup	140	2	13	4	1	12	7/na	45	20	na
Vanilla Ice Cream Sandwiches (Atkins)	1 serving	150	5	15	4	1	10	5/na	25	80	na

189

Food	Serving	Cal	Prot (g)	Carb (g)	Fiber (g)	Sugars (g)	Total Fat (g)	Sat/Trans Fat (g)	Chol (g)	Sod (mg)	GI
Vanilla, light, no sugar added	½ cup	105	3	14.5	.5	4	5	3/na	18	65	na
Vanilla Ice Cream Sandwiches (Atkins)	1 bar	140	3	12	4	1	16	12/na	30	25	na
Vanilla, soft-serve, ice milk	½ cup	164	4	24	0	na	6	4/na	28	92	na
Vanilla ice cream bar w/dark chocolate coating	1 bar	166	2	12	0	9	12	7/na	14	34	na
JAM, SUGAR, SYRUP, AND SWEETENERS											
Jams											
Apple butter	1 tbsp	29	t	7	t	6	0	0/0	0	1	na
Jams and preserves	1 tbsp	56	t	14	t	10	t	t/0	0	6	65
Jams and preserves	1 packet	39	t	10	t	7	t	t/0	0	4	65
Jams and preserves, dietetic	1 tbsp	18	t	7.5	t	5	t	t/0	0	0	30
Jam, apricot	1 tbsp	48	t	13	t	na	t	t/0	0	8	55

190

Food	Serving	Cal	Prot (g)	Carb (g)	Fiber (g)	Sugars (g)	Total Fat (g)	Sat/Trans Fat (g)	Chol (g)	Sod (mg)	GI
Jam, apricot	1 packet	34	t	9	t	na	t	t/0	0	6	55
Jam, strawberry	1 tbsp	0	0	0	0	0	0	t/0	0	0	51
Jellies, all types	1 tbsp	54	t	13	t	8	t	t/0	0	5	65
Jellies, all types	1 packet	40	t	10	t	6	t	t/0	0	4	65
Jelly, grape	1 tbsp	0	0	0	0	0	0	t/0	0	0	65
Orange marmalade	1 tbsp	49	t	13	0	na	0	0/0	0	11	48
Orange marmalade	1 packet	34	t	9	0	na	0	0/0	0	8	48
Strawberry spread, all-fruit	1 tbsp	42	t	10	na	8	0	0/0	0	4	55
Sugar											
Brown, unpacked	3 tsp	34	0	12	0	12	0	0/0	0	4	na
Maple	3 tsp	32	t	8	0	8	t	t/0	0	1	na
Powdered	3 tsp	29	0	7	0	7	t	t/0	0	0	na

Food	Serving	Cal	Prot (g)	Carb (g)	Fiber (g)	Sugars (g)	Total Fat (g)	Sat/Trans Fat (g)	Chol (g)	Sod (mg)	GI
White	1 lump (2 cubes)	19	0	5	0	5	0	0/0	0	0	58
White	1 packet	23	0	6	0	6	0	0/0	0	0	58
White	3 tsp	49	0	13	0	13	0	0/0	0	0	58
Syrups											
Blends, cane and 15% maple	1 tbsp	56	t	13	0	13	t	t/0	0	21	na
Blends, corn, refiner, and sugar	1 tbsp	64	0	17	0	17	0	0/0	0	14	na
Chocolate fudge-type syrup	2 tbsp	133	2	24	1	16	3	1.5/0	1	131	na
Chocolate lite (Hershey's)	2 tbsp	50	t	12	0	10	t	0/0	0	35	na
Corn, dark	1 tbsp	56	0	15	0	5	0	0/0	0	31	na
Corn, high fructose	1 tbsp	53	0	14	0	5	0	0/0	0	0	na
Corn, light	1 tbsp	56	0	17	0	6	0	0/0	0	24	na
Fruit syrup	1 tbsp	53	0	13	0	9	0	0/0	0	7	na
Honey, strained or extracted	1 tbsp	64	t	17	0	17	0	0/0	0	1	na

Food	Serving	Cal	Prot (g)	Carb (g)	Fiber (g)	Sugars (g)	Total Fat (g)	Sat/Trans Fat (g)	Chol (g)	Sod (mg)	GI
Honey, sugar-free	1 tbsp	50	0	17	0	0	0	0/0	0	0	na
Malt	1 tbsp	76	0	17	0	17	0	0/0	0	8	na
Maple syrup	1 tbsp	52	0	13	0	12	t	t/0	0	2	54
Molasses	1 tbsp	58	0	15	0	11	0	0/0	0	7	na
Pancake, regular	1 tbsp	57	0	12	0	6	0	0/0	0	17	na
Pancake, w/butter	1 tbsp	59	0	15	0	na	t	t/0	1	20	na
Pancake, w/2% pancake syrup	1 tbsp	53	0	14	0	8	t	t/0	0	12	na
Sorghum	1 tbsp	61	0	15	0	15	0	0/0	0	2	na
Syrup, dietetic	1 tbsp	6	t	7	t	0	0	0/0	0	3	na

Food	Serving	Cal	Prot (g)	Carb (g)	Fiber (g)	Sugars (g)	Total Fat (g)	Sat/Trans Fat (g)	Chol (mg)	Sod (mg)
LAMB										
Ground, broiled	4 oz	320	28	0	0	0	22	9/0	108	92
Leg, shank half, lean only, trimmed to ¼" fat, choice, roasted	4 oz	204	32	0	0	0	7.5	3/0	99	75
Leg, shank half, lean and fat, trimmed to ¼" fat, choice, roasted	4 oz	246	30	0	0	0	13	5/0	102	74
Leg, sirloin half, lean only, trimmed to ¼" fat, choice, roasted	4 oz	231	32	0	0	0	10	4/0	104	80
Leg, whole (shank and sirloin), lean only, trimmed to ¼" fat, choice, roasted	4 oz	216	32	0	0	0	9	3/0	101	77
Loin, lean only, trimmed to ¼" fat, choice, broiled	4 oz	245	34	0	0	0	11	4/0	108	95
Loin, lean only, trimmed to ¼" fat, choice, roasted	4 oz	229	30	0	0	0	11	4/0	99	75

Food	Serving	Cal	Prot (g)	Carb (g)	Fiber (g)	Sugars (g)	Total Fat (g)	Sat/Trans Fat (g)	Chol (mg)	Sod (mg)
Retail cuts, lean and fat, trimmed to 1/8" fat, choice, cooked	4 oz	307	29	0	0	0	20	8/0	109	82
Rib, lean and fat, trimmed to 1/8" fat, choice, broiled	4 oz	385	26	0	0	0	30	13/0	111	87
Rib, lean and fat, trimmed to 1/8" fat, choice, roasted	4 oz	386	25	0	0	0	31	13/0	109	84
Rib, lean and fat, trimmed to 1/4" fat, choice, broiled	4 oz	409	25	0	0	0	34	14/0	112	86
Rib, lean and fat, trimmed to 1/4" fat, choice, roasted	4 oz	407	24	0	0	0	34	14/0	110	83
Shoulder/arm, lean only, trimmed to 1/4" fat, choice, broiled	4 oz	227	31	0	0	0	10	4/0	104	93
Shoulder/arm, lean only, trimmed to 1/4" fat, choice, roasted	4 oz	218	29	0	0	0	10	4/0	97	76
Shoulder, whole (arm and shoulder), lean only, trimmed to 1/4" fat, choice, broiled	4 oz	238	31	0	0	0	12	4/0	105	94

Food	Serving	Cal	Prot (g)	Carb (g)	Fiber (g)	Sugars (g)	Total Fat (g)	Sat/Trans Fat (g)	Chol (mg)	Sod (mg)
Shoulder, whole (arm and shoulder), lean only, trimmed to ¼" fat, choice, broiled	4 oz	231	28	0	0	0	12	5/0	99	77
Sirloin chop, lean only, broiled	4 oz	213	31	0	0	0	9	4/0	96	75
LUNCHMEATS, BACON, AND SAUSAGE										
Bacon, Canadian-style, grilled	2 slices	87	11	1	0	0	4	1/0	27	727
Bacon, fried, drained	3 strips	108	6	t	0	t	9	3/0	16	301
Bacon, meatless	2 strips	31	1	1	t	na	3	1/0	0	147
Bacon, turkey	1 serving	35	2	t	0	t	3	1/0	13	170
Beerwurst, beef	1 slice	76	3	t	0	na	7	3/0	14	236
Beerwurst, pork	1 slice	55	3	.5	0	na	4	1.5/0	14	285
Blood sausage	1 slice	94	4	0	0	0	9	3/0	30	30
Bologna, fat-free	1 serving	22	3.5	2	0	1	t	t/0	7	274
Bologna, beef	1 slice	87	3	t	0	na	8	3/t	16	275

Food	Serving	Cal	Prot (g)	Carb (g)	Fiber (g)	Sugars (g)	Total Fat (g)	Sat/Trans Fat (g)	Chol (mg)	Sod (mg)
Bologna, beef, Lebanon	1 slice	112	11	t	0	1.5	7.5	3/t	35	773
Bologna, pork	1 slice	69	4	t	0	na	6	2/t	17	332
Bologna, pork and beef	1 slice	87	3	1	0	1	8	3/t	15	285
Bologna, pork and turkey, lite	2 slices	118	7	2	0	0	9	3/t	44	401
Bologna, turkey	2 slices	113	8	t	0	na	9	3/t	56	500
Bratwurst, beef and pork, smoked	2 oz	168	7	1.5	0	0	15	3/na	44	480
Bratwurst, pork, cooked	1 link	256	12	2	0	na	22	8/na	51	473
Bratwurst, pork, beef and turkey, lite, smoked	2 oz	129	9	3	0	1	9	3/na	37	648
Bratwurst, veal, cooked	2 oz	194	8	0	0	0	18	8.5/na	45	34
Braunschweiger	1 slice	65	2.5	.5	0	0	6	2/na	28	206
Breakfast links, turkey sausage	2 links	129	9	1	0	0	10	2/na	34	328
Chicken, smoked	2 oz	94	10	t	0	na	6	1/na	30	544
Chicken, white, oven-roasted (Louis Rich)	1 serving	36	5	1	0	t	2	t/0	17	335

197

Food	Serving	Cal	Prot (g)	Carb (g)	Fiber (g)	Sugars (g)	Total Fat (g)	Sat/Trans Fat (g)	Chol (mg)	Sod (mg)
Chicken, white, oven-roasted deluxe (Louis Rich)	1 serving	28	5	1	0	t	t	t/0	14	333
Chicken breast Classic Baked (Louis Rich)	2 slices	43	9	2	0	t	t	t/0	23	502
Chicken breast, honey glazed (Oscar Mayer)	2 slices	28	5	1	0	1	t	t/0	14	374
Chicken breast, oven-roasted, fat-free	2 slices	33	7	1	0	t	t	t/0	16	457
Chicken breast, smoked, mesquite flavor	2 slices	34	7	1	0	t	t	t/0	15	437
Ham, extra lean	2 slices	73	11	t	0	na	3	1/0	26	800
Ham, 96% fat-free (Oscar Mayer)	2 slices	44	7	1	0	t	1	t/0	20	521
Hot smoked turkey sausage	2 oz	88	8	3	.5	2	5	2/0	30	520
Knockwurst	1 link	221	8	2	0	na	20	7/0	43	670
Liverwurst	1 slice	59	2.5	t	0	na	5	2/0	28	155
Meatless sausage	1 link	64	5	2	1	na	5	1/0	0	222

Food	Serving	Cal	Prot (g)	Carb (g)	Fiber (g)	Sugars (g)	Total Fat (g)	Sat/Trans Fat (g)	Chol (mg)	Sod (mg)
Meatless sausage	1 patty	97	7	4	1	na	7	1/0	0	337
Salami, turkey	2 slices	82	8	t	0	t	5	t/0	42	562
Pork sausage links	2 links	165	8	.5	0	t	15	5/na	37	401
Pork sausage patties	2 patties	199	11	.5	0	na	17	6/na	45	699
Pork sausage, Italian	1 link	216	13	1	0	na	17	6/na	52	618
Pork sausage, Polish	1 sausage	740	32	4	0	na	65	23/na	159	1,989
Pork and beef sausage, cooked	2 links	103	4	1	0	na	9	3/na	18	209
Pork and beef sausage, cooked	2 patties	214	7.5	1.5	0	na	20	7/na	38	435
Salami, beef	2 slices	204	10	t	0	t	18	5/na	39	930
Salami, beef and pork	2 slices	115	6	1	0	na	9	4/na	30	490
Smoked sausage, turkey	1 serving	90	8	2	0	2	6	1/0	37	530

Food	Serving	Cal	Prot (g)	Carb (g)	Fiber (g)	Sugars (g)	Total Fat (g)	Sat/Trans Fat (g)	Chol (mg)	Sod (mg)
Smokies Sausage Little (pork, turkey) (Oscar Mayer)	2 links	54	2	t	0	t	5	2/0	12	184
Summer sausage, w/ cheese	2 oz	242	11	1	t	t	21.5	6/0	50	841
Swisswurst, pork and beef, w/Swiss cheese, smoked	1 serving (2.7 oz)	236	10	1	0	0	21	8/0	47	637
Turkey breast, oven-roasted, fat-free (Louis Rich)	2 slices	101	21	2	0	t	t	t/0	45	1,318
Turkey breast, smoked (Oscar Mayer)	2 slices	21	4	1	0	t	t	t/0	8	285
Turkey breast and white turkey, smoked (Louis Rich)	2 slices	56	10	1	0	t	1	t/0	24	514
Turkey ham	2 slices	64	10	t	0	t	2	t/0	38	632
Turkey ham, cured turkey thigh meat	2 slices	73	11	t	0	0	3	1/0	32	32
Vienna sausage	7 links	315	12	2	0	0	28.5	10.5/0	59	1,077

Food	Serving	Cal	Prot (g)	Carb (g)	Fiber (g)	Sugars (g)	Total Fat (g)	Sat/Trans Fat (g)	Chol (g)	Sod (mg)	GI
MEAL REPLACEMENT SUPPLEMENTS											
Bars											
Chocolate bar (Balance)	1 bar	200	14	22	1	18	6	4/na	5	230	25
Chocolate Fudge—CarbWell (Balance)	1 bar	190	14	23	2	1	6	4/0	5	190	na
Chocolate Chip (Clif Bar)	1 bar	250	10	45	5	21	5	2/0	0	150	68
Energy bar, all flavors (Gatorade)	1 bar (2.3 oz)	255	7	47	1.5	21	5	1/0	0	170	na
Energy, sport, or breakfast bar, generic	1 medium bar	202	12	27	2	0	5	3/na	2	130	na
Energy, sport, or breakfast bar, generic	1 small bar	140	6	22	3.5	0	4	2/na	2	75	na
Peanut butter (Met-Rx)	1 bar (3.5 oz)	344	27	50	na	29	4	1	10	135	55

Food	Serving	Cal	Prot (g)	Carb (g)	Fiber (g)	Sugars (g)	Total Fat (g)	Sat/Trans Fat (g)	Chol (g)	Sod (mg)	GI
Peanut butter Nutrilite Positrim Food Bar	1 serving (2 bars)	210	8	26	0	18	9	2.5	3	170	na
Drinks											
Drink mix, Promax (Sport Pharma)	1 serving (2 scoops)	255	50	6	0	0	4	2/na	0	120	na
Drink mix, original (Met-Rx)	1 serving packet (2.5 oz)	251	38	19	0	3	3	2/na	15	370	na
Ensure, regular	1 can (8 fl oz)	250	9	40	0	18	6	.5/0	t	200	48
Ensure Fiber with FOS	1 can (8 fl oz)	250	9	42	3	12	6	.5/0	t	200	na
Ensure Plus, high protein	1 can (8 fl oz)	360	13	50	0	16	11	1/0	t	240	na

Food	Serving	Cal	Prot (g)	Carb (g)	Fiber (g)	Sugars (g)	Total Fat (g)	Sat/Trans Fat (g)	Chol (g)	Sod (mg)	GI
Equate Plus	1 can	350	9	47	t	18	11	1/0	t	240	na
Fruit juice mixable formula, powdered, not reconstituted	1 scoop	89	10	17	6	na	0	0/0	0	74	na
Milk-based liquid, high protein	1 cup	240	15	33	0	na	6	1/0	0	220	na
Positrim Drink Mix, not reconstituted (Amway Nutrilite)	1 packet	162	7	27	0	na	4	1/0	3	106	na
Reduced-calorie meal replacement shake, generic	1 can	220	11	38	4	33	3	t/0	5	220	na
Shake, isotonic liquid nutrition w/fiber (Jevity)	237 ml	250	10	37	3	na	8	na/na	na	220	na
Shake, isotonic liquid nutrition (Jevity)	1 can (8 fl oz)	261	8	36	na	na	8	na/na	na	220	48
Shake, RxFuel (TwinLab)	1 serving	250	1	62	na	na	0	0/0	na	na	na
Shake, vanilla (GeniSoy)	1 scoop, dry (1.2 oz)	128	14	18	0	13	0	0/0	na	180	na

Food	Serving	Cal	Prot (g)	Carb (g)	Fiber (g)	Sugars (g)	Total Fat (g)	Sat/Trans Fat (g)	Chol (g)	Sod (mg)	GI
Weight-loss shake, strawberries and cream (Equate)	1 can (11 fl oz)	230	9	47	na	34	2	1/na	10	370	na
MILK, CREAM, AND MILK PRODUCTS											
Milk and Milk Products											
Buttermilk, low-fat	1 cup	98	8	12	0	12	2	1/0	10	257	na
Chocolate milk	1 cup	208	8	26	2	24	8	5/0	30	150	24–42
Chocolate syrup, prepared w/ whole milk	1 cup	257	9	36	1	na	9	5	34	147	na
Dry milk, nonfat, instant	⅓ cup	82	8	12	0	0	t	t/0	4	125	na
Eggnog	1 cup	343	9	34	0	21	19	11/0	150	137	na
Eggnog-flavored mix, prepared w/whole milk	1 cup	261	8	39	1	34	8	5/0	33	163	na

Food	Serving	Cal	Prot (g)	Carb (g)	Fiber (g)	Sugars (g)	Total Fat (g)	Sat/Trans Fat (g)	Chol (g)	Sod (mg)	GI
Evaporated milk, canned, nonfat	½ cup	100	10	15	0	15	t	t/0	5	147	na
Hot cocoa, homemade	1 cup	193	10	29	2	24	6	4/t	20	128	na
Low-fat milk, 1%, protein fortified	1 cup	118	10	14	0	na	3	2/0	10	143	na
Low-fat milk, 1%, regular	1 cup	102	8	12	0	na	3	2/0	10	124	34
Malted drink mix, prepared w/whole milk	1 cup	236	9	30	t	18	9	5/na	34	172	45
Milk, canned, condensed, sweetened	½ cup	491	12	83	0	83	13	8	52	194	61
Milk substitutes, fluid, w/hydrogenated vegetable oils	1 cup	149	4	15	0	15	8	2/na	0	190	na
Nonfat milk (skim or fat-free)	1 cup	86	8	12	0	12	t	t/0	5	127	32
Reduced-fat milk, 2%	1 cup	122	8	12	0	na	5	3/0	20	122	34
Strawberry-flavored beverage mix, prepared w/whole milk	1 cup	234	8	33	0	na	8	5/0	32	128	na
Whole milk	1 cup	156	8	11	0	13	9	6/0	34	120	40

205

Food	Serving	Cal	Prot (g)	Carb (g)	Fiber (g)	Sugars (g)	Total Fat (g)	Sat/Trans Fat (g)	Chol (g)	Sod (mg)	GI
Cream											
Creamer, nondairy, w/hydrogenated vegetable oil and soy protein	1 tbsp	20	t	2	0	3	2	t/0	0	12	na
Creamer, nondairy, w/lauric acid oil and sodium caseinate	1 tbsp	20	t	2	0	na	2	1/0	0	12	na
Creamer, powdered, light	1 packet	13	0	2	0	2	.5	t/0	0	7	na
Half and Half	1 tbsp	20	t	1	0	t	2	1/0	6	6	0
Liquid, coffee or table	1 tbsp	29	t	1	0	t	3	2/0	10	6	0
Whipping, heavy	1 tbsp	52	t	t	0	t	6	3/0	21	6	0
Sour cream	1 tbsp	26	t	1	0	na	3	2/0	5	6	0
NUTS, SEEDS, AND NUT BUTTERS											
Nuts and Seeds											
Almonds, dry roasted, w/salt	1 tbsp	51	2	2	1	t	5	t/0	0	29	15
Almonds, dry roasted, w/o salt	1 tbsp	51	2	2	1	t	5	t/0	0	0	15

Food	Serving	Cal	Prot (g)	Carb (g)	Fiber (g)	Sugars (g)	Total Fat (g)	Sat/Trans Fat (g)	Chol (g)	Sod (mg)	GI
Almonds, honey roasted	1 tbsp	53	2	2.5	1	na	4	t/0	0	12	15
Almonds, oil roasted, w/salt	1 tbsp	60	2	2	1	t	5	t/na	0	33	15
Almonds, oil roasted, w/o salt	1 tbsp	60	2	2	1	t	5	t/na	0	0	15
Brazil nuts, dried	1 tbsp	57	1	1	.5	t	6	1/0	0	0	na
Cashews, dry roasted, w/salt	1 tbsp	49	1	3	t	t	4	1/0	0	55	27
Cashews, dry roasted, w/o salt	1 tbsp	49	1	3	t	t	4	1/0	0	1	25
Cashews, oil roasted, w/salt	1 tbsp	47	1	2	t	t	4	1/na	0	25	27
Cashews, oil roasted, w/o salt	1 tbsp	47	1	2	t	t	4	1/na	0	1	25
Coconut cream, canned	½ cup	284	4	12	3	9	26	23/0	0	74	na
Coconut meat, dried, not sweetened	1 tbsp	94	1	3	2	t	9	8/0	0	5	45
Coconut meat, dried, sweetened, flaked, canned	½ cup	171	1	16	2	t	12	11/0	0	8	na
Coconut meat, dried, sweetened, flaked, package	½ cup	175	1	18	2	na	12	11/0	0	95	na

207

Food	Serving	Cal	Prot (g)	Carb (g)	Fiber (g)	Sugars (g)	Total Fat (g)	Sat/Trans Fat (g)	Chol (g)	Sod (mg)	GI
Coconut meat, dried, sweetened, shredded	½ cup	233	1	22	2	20	16.5	15/0	0	122	na
Coconut milk, canned	1 cup	445	5	6	na	na	48	43/0	0	29	40
Flaxseeds, ground	1 tbsp	37	1	2	2	t	3	t/0	0	2	na
Flaxseeds, whole	1 tbsp	55	2	3	3	t	4	t/0	0	3	na
Hazelnuts or filberts	1 tbsp	53	1	1	1	t	5	t/0	0	0	15
Hickory nuts, dried	1 tbsp	49	1	1	.5	na	5	.5/0	0	0	15
Macadamia nuts, dry roasted, w/salt	1 tbsp	60	1	1	1	t	6	1/0	0	22	na
Macadamia nuts, dry roasted, w/o salt	1 tbsp	60	1	1	1	t	6	1/0	0	0	na
Mixed nuts, dry roasted, w/salt	1 tbsp	51	1	2	1	na	4	1/0	0	57	24
Mixed nuts, dry roasted, w/o salt	1 tbsp	51	1	2	1	na	4	1/0	0	1	24
Mixed nuts, oil roasted, w/peanuts, w/salt	1 tbsp	55	1	2	1	na	5	1/na	0	58	24
Mixed nuts, oil roasted, w/peanuts, w/o salt	1 tbsp	55	1	2	1	na	5	1/na	0	11	24

Food	Serving	Cal	Prot (g)	Carb (g)	Fiber (g)	Sugars (g)	Total Fat (g)	Sat/Trans Fat (g)	Chol (g)	Sod (mg)	GI
Mixed nuts, oil roasted, w/o peanuts, w/salt	1 tbsp	55	1	2	.5	t	5	1/0	0	63	24
Mixed nuts, oil roasted, w/o peanuts, w/o salt	1 tbsp	55	1	2	.5	t	5	1/0	0	1	24
Peanuts, all types, boiled, w/salt	½ cup	286	12	19	8	t	20	3/0	0	676	15
Peanuts, all types, dry roasted, w/salt	10 peanuts	59	2	2	1	t	5	1/0	0	81	15
Peanuts, all types, dry roasted, w/o salt	10 peanuts	59	2	2	1	t	5	1/0	0	1	15
Peanuts, oil roasted, w/salt	10 peanuts	54	2.5	1	1	t	5	1/na	0	29	15
Peanuts, oil roasted, w/o salt	10 peanuts	54	2.5	1	1	t	5	1/na	0	1	15
Pecans	1 tbsp	47	1	1	1	t	5	t/0	0	0	na
Pecans, oil roasted, w/salt	1 tbsp	49	1	1	1	t	5	t/na	0	27	na
Pistachio nuts, dry roasted, w/salt	1 tbsp	45	2	2	1	1	4	t/0	0	32	na

Food	Serving	Cal	Prot (g)	Carb (g)	Fiber (g)	Sugars (g)	Total Fat (g)	Sat/Trans Fat (g)	Chol (g)	Sod (mg)	GI
Pistachio nuts, dry roasted, w/o salt	1 tbsp	45	2	2	1	1	4	t/0	0	1	na
Pumpkin and squash seeds, whole, roasted, w/salt	1 oz (85 seeds)	126	5	15	na	na	5.5	1/0	0	163	25
Pumpkin and squash seeds, whole, roasted, w/o salt	1 oz (85 seeds)	126	5	15	na	na	5.5	1/0	0	5	25
Sesame seeds, whole, roasted and toasted	1 oz	160	5	7	4	na	14	2/0	0	3	na
Sunflower seeds, dried	1 tbsp	57	2	2	1	na	5	.5/0	0	0	35
Sunflower seeds, dry roasted, w/salt	1 tbsp	52	2	2	1	na	5	.5/0	0	70	35
Sunflower seeds, dry roasted, w/o salt	1 tbsp	52	2	2	1	na	5	.5/0	0	0	35
Sunflower seeds, oil roasted, w/salt	1 tbsp	58	2	1	1	na	5	.5/na	0	57	35
Sunflower seeds, oil roasted, w/o salt	1 tbsp	58	2	1	1	na	5	.5/na	0	0	35

Food	Serving	Cal	Prot (g)	Carb (g)	Fiber (g)	Sugars (g)	Total Fat (g)	Sat/Trans Fat (g)	Chol (g)	Sod (mg)	GI
Sunflower seeds, toasted, w/salt	1 tbsp	58	2	2	1	na	5	.5/na	0	57	35
Trail mix, tropical	1 cup	570	9	92	0	na	24	12	0	14	na
Trail mix, regular, w/chocolate chips, salted nuts and seeds	1 cup	707	21	66	0	na	47	9/na	6	177	24
Trail mix, regular, w/chocolate chips, unsalted nuts and seeds	1 cup	707	21	66	0	na	47	9/na	6	39	24
Walnuts, English	1 tbsp	41	1	1	t	t	4	4/0	0	0	15
Nut Butters											
Almond butter, w/salt	1 tbsp	101	2	3	1	1	9	1/0	0	72	na
Almond butter, w/o salt	1 tbsp	101	2	3	1	1	9	1/0	0	2	na
Cashew butter, w/salt	1 tbsp	94	3	4	t	na	8	1.5/na	0	98	na
Cashew butter, w/o salt	1 tbsp	94	3	4	t	na	8	1.5/na	0	2	na
Nutella	2 tbsp	200	2	23	2	20	11	2/0	0	15	55
Peanut butter, chunk style, vitamin fortified	1 tbsp	94	4	3.5	1	3.5	8	1.5/0	0	73	40

Food	Serving	Cal	Prot (g)	Carb (g)	Fiber (g)	Sugars (g)	Total Fat (g)	Sat/Trans Fat (g)	Chol (g)	Sod (mg)	GI
Peanut butter, chunk style w/salt	1 tbsp	94	4	3.5	1	3	8	1/0	0	78	40
Peanut butter, chunk style w/o salt	1 tbsp	94	4	3.5	1	3	8	1/0	0	3	40
Peanut butter, reduced sodium	1 tbsp	101	4	3.5	1	1	8	1.5/0	0	32	40
Peanut butter, smooth style, w/salt	1 tbsp	94	4	3	1	3	8	1.5/0	0	73	40
Peanut butter, smooth style, w/o salt	1 tbsp	94	4	3	1	3	8	1.5/0	0	3	40
Peanut butter, smooth, reduced fat	1 tbsp	109	5	7	1	1.5	7	1/0	0	113	40
Peanut butter, smooth style, vitamin fortified	1 tbsp	95	4	3	1	1.5	8	1.5/0	0	67	40
Sesame butter (tahini)	1 tbsp	89	2.5	3	1.4	t	8	1/0	0	17	40

212

Food	Serving	Cal	Prot (g)	Carb (g)	Fiber (g)	Sugars (g)	Total Fat (g)	Sat/Trans Fat (g)	Chol (mg)	Sod (mg)
ORGAN MEATS										
Beef heart, simmered	4 oz	187	32	0	0	0	5	1.5/t	240	67
Beef kidneys, simmered	4 oz	179	31	0	0	0	5	1/t	811	107
Beef liver, braised	1 slice	130	20	3.5	0	0	3.5	1/t	269	54
Brain, beef, simmered	4 oz	181	13	0	0	0	14	3/0	2,328	136
Brain, beef, pan-fried	4 oz	222	14	0	0	0	18	4/0	2,261	179
Brain, pork, braised	4 oz	156	14	0	0	0	11	2/0	2,892	103
Giblets, fried	1 cup, chopped or diced	402	47	6	0	0	20	5/0	647	164
Pork heart, braised	1 heart	191	30	.5	0	0	6.5	2/0	285	45
Pork kidneys, braised	4 oz	171	29	0	0	0	5	2/0	544	91
Pork liver, braised	4 oz	187	29	4	0	0	5	1.5/0	402	56
Pork spleen, braised	4 oz	169	32	0	0	0	4	1/0	571	121
Sweetbread, braised	4 oz	362	25	0	0	0	28	10/0	333	131
Tripe, raw	4 oz	111	16	0	0	0	4	2/0	107	52

213

Food	Serving	Cal	Prot (g)	Carb (g)	Fiber (g)	Sugars (g)	Total Fat (g)	Sat/Trans Fat (g)	Chol (mg)	Sod (mg)
Tongue, beef, simmered	4 oz	321	25	t	0	0	24	10/0	121	68
Tongue, pork, simmered	4 oz	307	27	0	0	0	21	7/0	165	124
Veal liver, braised	4 oz	187	24.5	3	0	0	8	3/0	636	60
Veal spleen, braised	4 oz	146	27	0	0	0	3	1/0	507	66

Food	Serving	Cal	Prot (g)	Carb (g)	Fiber (g)	Sugars (g)	Total Fat (g)	Sat/Trans Fat (g)	Chol (mg)	Sod (mg)	GI
PANCAKES AND WAFFLES											
Pancakes											
Blueberry pancakes, prepared from recipe	1 pancake (4"dia.)	84	2	11	na	na	4	1/0	21	157	na
Blueberry pancakes, prepared from recipe	1 pancake (6"dia.)	171	5	22	na	na	7	2/0	43	317	na
Buttermilk mini pancakes, frozen, ready to microwave	1 serving	116	4	22	na	1	2	t/0	na	290	na
Buttermilk pancakes, prepared from recipe	1 pancake (4"dia.)	86	3	11	na	na	4	1/0	22	198	na
Buttermilk pancakes, prepared from recipe	1 pancake (6"dia.)	175	5	22	na	na	7	1/0	45	402	na
Plain pancakes, dry mix, prepared	1 pancake (4"dia.)	74	2	14	.5	na	1	t/0	5	239	na

215

Food	Serving	Cal	Prot (g)	Carb (g)	Fiber (g)	Sugars (g)	Total Fat (g)	Sat/Trans Fat (g)	Chol (mg)	Sod (mg)	GI
Plain pancakes, dry mix, prepared	1 pancake (6"dia.)	149	4	28	1	na	2	t/0	9	484	na
Plain pancakes, frozen, ready-to-heat	1 mini pancake	23	1	4	t	na	t	t/0	1	51	na
Plain pancakes, frozen, ready-to-heat	1 pancake (4"dia.)	94	2	18	1	4	1	t/0	4	209	na
Plain pancakes, frozen, ready-to-heat	1 pancake (6"dia.)	167	4	32	1	7	2	1	7	372	na
Plain pancakes, prepared from recipe	1 pancake (4"dia.)	86	2	11	na	na	4	1/0	22	167	na
Plain pancakes, prepared from recipe	1 pancake (6"dia.)	175	5	22	na	na	7	2/0	45	338	na

Food	Serving	Cal	Prot (g)	Carb (g)	Fiber (g)	Sugars (g)	Total Fat (g)	Sat/Trans Fat (g)	Chol (mg)	Sod (mg)	GI
Whole-wheat pancakes, dry mix, prepared	1 pancake (4"dia.)	92	4	13	1	na	3	1/0	27	252	na
Whole-wheat pancakes, dry mix, prepared	1 pancake (6"dia.)	268	11	38	4	na	8	2/0	79	738	na
Waffles											
Banana bread waffles	1 serving	212	5	32	2	5	7	1/0	0	280	76
Buttermilk waffles, frozen, ready-to-heat	1 waffle (4" square)	98	2	15	1	na	3	t/0	12	292	76
Buttermilk waffles, frozen, ready-to-heat, toasted	1 waffle (4" dia.)	87	2	13	1	na	3	t/0	8	260	76
Eggo Low-fat Blueberry Waffles (Kellogg's)	1 waffle (4" dia.)	83	2.5	15.5	t	1	1	t/0	9	155	na
Eggo Low-fat Homestyle Waffles (Kellogg's)	1 waffle (4" dia.)	83	2	15	1	3	1	t/0	0	207	na

217

Food	Serving	Cal	Prot (g)	Carb (g)	Fiber (g)	Sugars (g)	Total Fat (g)	Sat/Trans Fat (g)	Chol (mg)	Sod (mg)	GI
Eggo Low-fat Nutri-Grain Waffles (Kellogg's)	1 waffle (4" dia.)	71	2	14	1	2	1	t/0	0	215	na
Frozen waffles	1 serving	197	5	30	na	na	6	1/0	12	563	76
Oat waffles	1 waffle (4" dia.)	69	2	13	1	1	1	t/0	0	135	na
Plain waffles	1 waffle (7" dia.)	218	6	25	na	na	11	2/0	52	383	76
PASTA AND NOODLES											
Alfredo egg noodles in creamy sauce, dry mix (Lipton)	1 serving	259	10	39	0	na	7	7/na	69	1,097	na
Chinese noodles, chow mein, cooked	½ cup	119	2	13	1	t	7	1	0	99	35
Corn pasta, cooked	½ cup	88	2	20	3	na	t	t	0	0	>70
Egg noodles, enriched, cooked	½ cup	106	4	20	1	t	1	t/t	26	6	<55
Egg noodles, spinach, enriched, cooked	½ cup	106	4	19	2	t	1	t/t	26	10	<55

218

Food	Serving	Cal	Prot (g)	Carb (g)	Fiber (g)	Sugars (g)	Total Fat (g)	Sat/Trans Fat (g)	Chol (mg)	Sod (mg)	GI
Fresh, refrigerated, plain	½ cup	149	6	28	na	na	1	t/0	38	7	58
Homemade, made w/o egg	½ cup	141	5	29	na	na	1	t/0	0	84	58
Japanese noodles, soba, cooked	½ cup	56	3	12	na	na	t	t/0	0	34	na
Japanese noodles, somen, cooked	½ cup	115	4	24	na	na	t	t/0	0	142	na
Macaroni, elbow	½ cup	99	3	20	1	t	t	t/0	0	1	47
Macaroni, elbow, whole wheat, cooked	½ cup	87	4	19	2	t	t	t/0	0	2	47
Macaroni, spiral	½ cup	94	3	19	1	t	t	t/0	0	1	47
Macaroni, shells	½ cup	81	3	16	1	t	t	t/0	0	1	47
Spaghetti, w/salt	½ cup	99	3	20	1	na	t	t/0	0	70	58
Spinach pasta, refrigerated, cooked	½ cup	148	6	29	na	na	1	t/0	38	7	na
Spinach spaghetti, cooked	½ cup	91	3	18	na	na	t	t/0	0	10	na

219

Food	Serving	Cal	Prot (g)	Carb (g)	Fiber (g)	Sugars (g)	Total Fat (g)	Sat/Trans Fat (g)	Chol (mg)	Sod (mg)	GI
Tortellini, pasta w/cheese filling	¾ cup	249	11	38	1.5	1	6	3/0	34	279	50
Whole-wheat spaghetti	½ cup	87	4	19	3	na	t	t/0	0	2	32
PICKLES AND OLIVES											
Pickles											
Dill pickle	1 spear	5	t	1	t	na	t	t/0	0	385	15
Dill pickle, chopped	½ cup	13	t	3	1	na	t	t/0	0	917	15
Dill pickle, large (4" long)	1 pickle	24	1	6	2	na	t	t/0	0	1,731	15
Dill pickle, medium (3¾" long)	1 pickle	12	t	3	1	na	t	t/0	0	833	15
Dill pickle, small	1 pickle	7	t	2	t	na	t	t/0	0	474	15
Sour pickle	1 spear	3	t	1	t	na	t	t/0	0	362	15
Sour pickle, chopped	½ cup	36	t	2	1	na	t	t/0	0	936	15
Sour pickle, large (4" long)	1 pickle	15	t	3	2	na	t	t/0	0	1,631	15
Sour pickle, medium (3¾" long)	1 pickle	7	t	1	1	na	t	t/0	0	785	15

Food	Serving	Cal	Prot (g)	Carb (g)	Fiber (g)	Sugars (g)	Total Fat (g)	Sat/Trans Fat (g)	Chol (mg)	Sod (mg)	GI
Sour pickle, small	1 pickle	4	t	1	t	na	t	t/0	0	447	15
Sweet pickle (Gherkin)	1 spear	23	t	6	t	na	t	t/0	0	188	na
Sweet pickle, chopped	½ cup	94	t	25	1	na	t	t/0	0	751	na
Sweet pickle (Gherkin), large (4" long)	1 pickle	41	t	11	t	na	t	t/0	0	329	na
Sweet pickle (Gherkin), medium (2¾" long)	1 pickle	29	t	8	t	na	t	t/0	0	235	na
Sweet pickle (Gherkin), midget (2⅛" long)	1 pickle	7	t	2	t	na	t	t/0	0	56	na
Sweet pickle (Gherkin), small (2½" long)	1 pickle	18	t	5	t	na	t	t/0	0	141	na
Olives											
Olive, green	5 olives	23	0	t	na	na	2.5	t/0	0	na	15
Olives, ripe, canned, colossal	1 olive	12	t	1	t	na	1	t/0	0	135	15
Olives, ripe, canned, jumbo	1 olive	7	t	t	t	na	1	t/0	0	75	15

Food	Serving	Cal	Prot (g)	Carb (g)	Fiber (g)	Sugars (g)	Total Fat (g)	Sat/Trans Fat (g)	Chol (mg)	Sod (mg)	GI
Olives, ripe, canned, large	1 olive	5	t	t	t	na	t	t/0	0	38	15
Olives, ripe, canned, small	1 olive	4	t	t	t	na	t	t/0	0	28	15
PIZZA											
Cheese Pizza, classic hand-tossed crust	1 slice	272	12	37	1.5	4	9	4/na	14	507	na
Cheese Pizza, original round, regular crust (Little Caesar's)	1 slice	236	12	28	1.5	2	8.5	4/na	21	404	na
Cheese Pizza, original crust (Papa John's)	1 slice	304	13	38	2	6	11	5/na	22	676	na
Cheese Pizza, regular crust (Pizza Hut)	1 slice	271	12	32	1	3	11	4/na	26	632	na
Cheese, slice	1 slice	140	8	21	0	4	3	1.5/na	9	336	60
Cheese, meat, and vegetables, slice	1 slice	184	13	21	na	5	5	1.5/na	21	382	36
Cheese, sausage, pepperoni, and onions, frozen	1 serving	337	12	32	na	na	18	6/na	25	704	36

Food	Serving	Cal	Prot (g)	Carb (g)	Fiber (g)	Sugars (g)	Total Fat (g)	Sat/Trans Fat (g)	Chol (mg)	Sod (mg)	GI
Crispy crust pepperoni, frozen	1 serving	364	13	35	na	na	19	4/na	12	973	na
Deep dish sausage pizza, frozen	1 serving	391	12	41	na	na	20	6/na	16	830	na
French bread pizza w/sausage and pepperoni, frozen	1 serving	448	18	44	2.5	na	22	7/na	37	860	na
French bread pizza w/sausage, pepperoni, and mushrooms, frozen	1 serving	429	16	44	3.5	na	21	6/na	33	840	na
Meat and Vegetable Pizza, regular crust (Little Caesar's)	1 slice	279	14	27	2	2	13	5/na	36	665	na
Mexican-Style pizza, frozen	1 serving	437	14	43	na	na	23	8/na	28	756	na
Pepperoni Pizza, classic hand-tossed crust (Domino's)	1 slice	324	14	39	2	4	13	5/na	26	608	na
Pepperoni, frozen	1 serving	400	16	36	2	na	21	7/na	34	879	na

Food	Serving	Cal	Prot (g)	Carb (g)	Fiber (g)	Sugars (g)	Total Fat (g)	Sat/Trans Fat (g)	Chol (mg)	Sod (mg)	GI
Pepperoni Pizza, original round, regular crust (Little Caesar's)	1 slice	246	12	28	2	4	9.5	4/na	25	466	na
Pizza snacks, hamburger, frozen	1 serving	231	9	26	na	na	10	na/na	na	417	na
Pizza snacks, pepperoni, frozen	1 serving	385	14	39	2	na	19	5/na	31	866	na
Pizza snacks, sausage, frozen	1 serving	351	14	40	3	na	15	3/na	24	632	na
Sausage, green and red peppers, mushroom, frozen	1 serving	386	17	33	na	na	21	8/na	37	765	36
Sausage and mushroom pizza, frozen	1 serving	306	14	31	na	na	14	5/na	26	718	36
Sausage, mushrooms, and pepperoni, frozen	1 serving	344	14	32	na	na	18	6/na	23	738	36

Food	Serving	Cal	Prot (g)	Carb (g)	Fiber (g)	Sugars (g)	Total Fat (g)	Sat/Trans Fat (g)	Chol (mg)	Sod (mg)	GI
Sausage and pepperoni, frozen	1 serving	348	17	30	na	na	17	7/na	44	708	na
Super Supreme Pizza, regular crust (Pizza Hut)	1 slice	305	14	32	3	8	14	5/na	34	809	na
The Works Pizza, original crust (Papa John's)	1 slice	367	16	41	4	7	16	6/na	32	872	na

Food	Serving	Cal	Prot (g)	Carb (g)	Fiber (g)	Sugars (g)	Total Fat (g)	Sat/Trans Fat (g)	Chol (mg)	Sod (mg)
PORK										
Boston blade, roasted	4 oz	304	26	0	0	0	21	8/0	96	76
Center loin chop, w/bone, lean only, braised	4 oz edible portion	229	34	0	0	0	9	3/0	96	70
Center loin chop, w/bone, lean only, broiled	4 oz edible portion	229	34	0	0	0	9	3/0	93	68
Cutlet, cooked	4 oz	284	32	0	0	0	17	6/0	96	64
Ground, cooked	4 oz	336	33	0	0	0	34	12/0	108	84
Ham, cured, whole, roasted	4 oz	275	24	0	0	0	19	7/0	70	1,345
Ham, patties, grilled	1 patty, cooked	205	8	1	0	0	19	7/0	43	638
Loin blade (chops), bone-in, lean and fat only, braised	4 oz	366	25	0	0	0	29	11/0	96	62
Loin blade (chops), bone-in, lean and fat only, broiled	4 oz	363	25	0	0	0	28	11/0	97	79

Food	Serving	Cal	Prot (g)	Carb (g)	Fiber (g)	Sugars (g)	Total Fat (g)	Sat/Trans Fat (g)	Chol (mg)	Sod (mg)
Loin blade (chops), bone-in, lean and fat only, pan-fried	4 oz	388	24	0	0	0	31	12/0	96	76
Loin blade (chops), bone-in, lean and fat only, roasted	4 oz	366	27	0	0	0	28	10/0	105	34
Loin, country-style ribs, lean and fat only, braised	4 oz	335	27	0	0	0	24	9/0	99	67
Loin, country-style ribs, lean and fat only, roasted	4 oz	372	27	0	0	0	29	10/0	104	59
Shoulder, arm picnic, lean and fat only, braised	4 oz	373	32	0	0	0	26	10/0	124	100
Shoulder, arm picnic, lean and fat only, roasted	4 oz	359	27	0	0	0	27	10/0	107	79
Shoulder, blade roll, lean and fat only, roasted	4 oz	325	20	t	0	na	27	9/0	76	1,103
Sirloin chop, w/bone, lean only, braised	4 oz edible portion	223	31	0	0	0	10	4/0	92	60

Food	Serving	Cal	Prot (g)	Carb (g)	Fiber (g)	Sugars (g)	Total Fat (g)	Sat/Trans Fat (g)	Chol (mg)	Sod (mg)
Sirloin chop, boneless, lean only, broiled	4 oz	219	35	0	0	0	8	3/0	104	63
Sirloin roast, boneless, lean only, roasted	4 oz	224	33	0	0	0	9	3/0	97	63
Spareribs, cooked	4 oz	448	33	0	0	0	34	12/0	136	104
Tenderloin, lean only, broiled	4 oz	212	34	0	0	0	7	2.5/0	107	74
Tenderloin, lean only, roasted	4 oz	186	32	0	0	0	5.5	2/0	90	63
Tenderloin, lean and fat, broiled	4 oz	228	34	0	0	0	9	3/0	107	75
Top loin chop, boneless, lean only, braised	4 oz	229	33	0	0	0	10	4/0	83	48
Top loin chop, boneless, lean only, braised	4 oz	230	35	0	0	0	9	3/0	91	74

Food	Serving	Cal	Prot (g)	Carb (g)	Fiber (g)	Sugars (g)	Total Fat (g)	Sat/Trans Fat (g)	Chol (g)	Sod (mg)	GI
PUDDINGS											
Banana, dry mix, instant	1 portion makes 1/2 cup	92	0	23	0	15	t	t/0	0	375	na
Banana, dry mix, instant, w/added oil	1 portion makes 1/2 cup	97	0	22	0	na	1	t/0	0	375	na
Banana, dry mix, regular	1 portion makes 1/2 cup	83	0	20	t	16	t	t/0	0	173	na
Banana, dry mix, regular, w/added oil	1 portion makes 1/2 cup	85	0	19	t	na	1	t/0	0	173	na
Banana, ready-to-eat	1 can (5 oz)	180	3	30	t	na	5	1/0	0	278	na
Chocolate, dry mix, instant	1 portion makes 1/2 cup	89	1	22	1	17	t	t/0	0	357	na

Food	Serving	Cal	Prot (g)	Carb (g)	Fiber (g)	Sugars (g)	Total Fat (g)	Sat/Trans Fat (g)	Chol (g)	Sod (mg)	GI
Chocolate, dry mix, regular	1 portion makes ½ cup	90	1	22	.5	11	1	t/0	0	88	na
Chocolate, ready-to-eat	1 can (5 oz)	189	4	32	1	25	6	1/0	4	183	na
Chocolate, ready-to-eat	1 snack size (4 oz)	150	3	26	1	20	5	1/0	3	146	na
Chocolate, sugar-free, reduced-calorie, cook and serve (Jello-O)	1 portion makes ½ cup	31	t	7.5	1	t	t	t/0	0	109	na
Chocolate, sugar-free, reduced-calorie, instant (Jello-O)	1 portion makes ½ cup	34	.5	8	1	t	t	t/0	0	318	na
Coconut cream, dry mix, instant	1 portion makes ½ cup	97	t	22	t	na	1	1/0	0	302	na
Coconut cream, dry mix, regular	1 portion makes ½ cup	98	t	22	t	16	1	1/0	0	260	na

Food	Serving	Cal	Prot (g)	Carb (g)	Fiber (g)	Sugars (g)	Total Fat (g)	Sat/Trans Fat (g)	Chol (g)	Sod (mg)	GI
Lemon, dry mix, instant	1 portion makes ½ cup	95	0	24	0	na	t	t/0	0	333	na
Lemon, dry mix, regular	1 portion makes ½ cup	76	t	19	0	na	t	t	0	106	na
Lemon, ready-to-eat	1 can (5 oz)	178	t	36	t	na	4	1	0	199	na
Rice, dry mix	1 portion makes ½ cup	102	1	25	t	na	t	t	0	99	na
Rice, ready-to-eat	1 can (5 oz)	231	3	31	t	na	11	2	1	121	na
Tapioca, dry milk	1 portion makes ½ cup	85	t	22	0	15	t	t	0	110	na
Tapioca, ready-to-eat	1 can (5 oz)	169	3	28	t	25	5	1	1	226	na

Food	Serving	Cal	Prot (g)	Carb (g)	Fiber (g)	Sugars (g)	Total Fat (g)	Sat/Trans Fat (g)	Chol (g)	Sod (mg)	GI
Tapioca, ready-to-eat	1 snack size (4 oz)	134	2	22	t	20	4	1/0	1	180	na
Vanilla, dry mix, instant	1 portion makes ½ cup	92	0	23	0	19	t	t/0	0	360	na
Vanilla, dry mix, regular	1 portion makes ½ cup	81	t	21	t	16	t	t/0	0	166	na
Vanilla, ready-to-eat	1 snack size (4 oz)	147	3	25	t	23	4	1/0	8	153	na
Vanilla, sugar-free, reduced-calorie, cook and serve (Jello-O)	1 portion makes ½ cup	21	t	5	t	t	t	t/0	0	113	na
Vanilla, sugar-free, reduced-calorie, instant (Jello-O)	1 portion makes ½ cup	26	t	6	t	t	t	t/0	0	332	na

Food	Serving	Cal	Prot (g)	Carb (g)	Fiber (g)	Sugars (g)	Total Fat (g)	Sat/Trans Fat (g)	Chol (g)	Sod (mg)	GI
SALAD DRESSINGS											
Blue cheese, regular	1 tbsp	60	1	2	0	na	6	1/0	5	230	is
Blue cheese, low-fat	2 tbsp	60	0	4	0	na	4	2/0	10	480	is
Caesar salad dressing, low-calorie	2 tbsp	32	0	6	0	4	2	0/0	0	324	is
Coleslaw dressing, reduced-fat	2 tbsp	112	0	14	0	14	6	2/0	8	544	is
French, regular	1 tbsp	69	t	3	0	3	7	2/0	0	219	is
French, diet, low-fat	2 tbsp	43	t	7	0	3	2	t/0	0	252	is
Italian, regular	1 tbsp	69	t	2	0	1	7	1/0	0	116	is
Italian, diet	2 tbsp	32	t	1	0	na	3	t/0	2	236	is
Italian, fat-free (Kraft)	2 tbsp	20	t	4	t	2	t	t/0	1	430	is
Italian, Light Done Right (Kraft)	2 tbsp	53	t	2	t	0	4	t/0	0	228	is
Italian, zesty (Kraft)	1 tbsp	54	t	1	t	1	6	1/0	0	253	is
Ranch, regular (Kraft)	1 tbsp	74	t	t	0	t	8	1/0	4	144	is
Ranch, fat-free (Kraft)	2 tbsp	48	t	11	t	2	t	t/0	0	354	is
Ranch, Light Done Right (Kraft)	2 tbsp	77	t	3	t	1	7	t/0	8	303	is
Russian, regular	1 tbsp	74	t	2	3	3	8	1/0	3	130	is

Food	Serving	Cal	Prot (g)	Carb (g)	Fiber (g)	Sugars (g)	Total Fat (g)	Sat/Trans Fat (g)	Chol (g)	Sod (mg)	GI
Russian, low-calorie	2 tbsp	45	t	9	t	3.5	1	t/0	2	278	is
Sesame seed dressing	1 tbsp	66	t	1	t	1	7	1/0	0	150	is
Thousand Island, regular	1 tbsp	60	t	2	0	2	6	1/0	4	112	is
Thousand Island, low-calorie, diet	2 tbsp	48	t	5	t	3	3	t/0	5	300	is
Vinaigrette, balsamic	1 tbsp	50	0	2	0	2	4.5	1/0	0	165	is
Vinaigrette, red wine	1 tbsp	45	t	1	na	na	4.5	na/0	na	na	is
SNACKS											
Chips and Popcorn											
Banana chips	1 oz	147	1	16	2	10	9	8/na	0	2	na
Popcorn, oil-popped	2 cups	110	2	13	2	na	6	1/na	0	194	na
Pork skins, barbecue flavor	1 oz	152	16	0	0	na	9	2/na	32	753	na
Pork skins, plain	1 oz	154	17	0	0	0	9	3/na	27	519	na
Potato chips, fat-free	¼ bag (6 oz)	215	5.5	48	4	2	t	0/0	0	365	na
Potato chips, reduced-fat	¼ bag (6 oz)	200	3	28	3	na	9	2/na	0	209	na

234

Food	Serving	Cal	Prot (g)	Carb (g)	Fiber (g)	Sugars (g)	Total Fat (g)	Sat/Trans Fat (g)	Chol (g)	Sod (mg)	GI
Sesame sticks, wheat-based, salted	1 oz	153	3	13	1	t	10	2/na	0	420	na
Tortilla chips, light	20 chips	149	3	24	2	t	5	1/0	1	321	na
Tortilla chips, low-fat, unsalted	25 grams	104	3	20	1	t	1.5	t/0	0	4	na
Tortilla chips, low-fat, nacho cheese	25 grams	101	2	21	1	t	1	t/0	1	198	na
Pretzels											
Plain pretzel, hard, w/salt	10 twists	229	5	48	2	na	2/t	na	0	1,029	na
Plain pretzel, hard, w/o salt	10 twists	229	5	48	2	na	2/t	na	0	173	na
Pretzels, soft	1 large (143 grams)	483	12	99	2	0	4/1	na	4	2,008	na
Whole-wheat pretzel, hard	2 oz	206	6	46	4	na	1/t	na	0	116	na
SOUPS											
Bean w/frankfurters, canned, prepared w/water	1 cup (8 fl oz)	188	10	22	na	na	7	2	13	1,093	na
Bean w/ham, chunky, ready-to-serve	1 cup (8 fl oz)	231	13	27	11	na	9	3	22	972	na

235

Food	Serving	Cal	Prot (g)	Carb (g)	Fiber (g)	Sugars (g)	Total Fat (g)	Sat/Trans Fat (g)	Chol (g)	Sod (mg)	GI
Bean w/pork, canned, prepared w/water	1 cup (8 fl oz)	172	8	23	9	na	6	2	3	951	na
Beef broth or bouillon, canned, ready-to-serve	1 cup	17	3	t	0	na	1	t	0	782	na
Beef broth or bouillon, powder, prepared w/water	1 cup	20	1	2	0	na	1	t	0	1,362	na
Beef broth, cube, prepared w/water	1 cup	7	1	1	0	na	t	t	0	1,157	na
Beef w/country vegetables, chunky, ready-to-serve	1 serving	153	12	16	0	na	4	1	24	868	na
Beef, chunky, ready-to-serve	1 cup (8 fl oz)	170	12	20	1	na	5	3	14	866	na
Beef mushroom, canned, prepared w/water	1 cup	73	6	6	t	na	3	1	0	942	na
Beef noodle, canned, prepared w/water	1 cup	83	5	9	t	na	3	1	5	952	na
Beef noodle, dehydrated, prepared w/water	1 packet	30	2	4	1	na	1	t	2	776	na

236

Food	Serving	Cal	Prot (g)	Carb (g)	Fiber (g)	Sugars (g)	Total Fat (g)	Sat/Trans Fat (g)	Chol (g)	Sod (mg)	GI
Black bean, canned, prepared w/water	1 cup	116	6	20	5	na	2	t	0	1,198	64
Cauliflower, dehydrated, prepared w/water	1 cup	69	3	11	na	na	2	t	0	842	na
Cheese, canned, prepared w/milk	1 cup (8 fl oz)	231	10	16	1	na	14	9	48	1,019	na
Cheese, canned, prepared w/water	1 cup (8 fl oz)	156	5	11	1	na	10	7	30	958	na
Chicken broth, canned, prepared w/water	1 cup	39	5	1	0	na	1	t	0	776	na
Chicken broth, cube, prepared w/water	1 cup	12	1	2	na	na	t	t	0	792	na
Chicken broth or bouillion, dehydrated, prepared w/water	1 packet	16	1	1	0	na	1	t	0	1,113	na
Chicken, chunky, ready-to-serve	1 cup (8 fl oz)	178	13	17	2	na	7	2	30	889	na
Chicken corn chowder, chunky, ready-to-serve	1 serving	238	7	18	2	na	15	4	26	718	na

237

Food	Serving	Cal	Prot (g)	Carb (g)	Fiber (g)	Sugars (g)	Total Fat (g)	Sat/Trans Fat (g)	Chol (g)	Sod (mg)	GI
Chicken gumbo, canned, prepared w/water	1 cup	56	3	8	2	na	1	t	5	954	na
Chicken, mushroom chowder, chunky, ready-to-serve	1 serving	192	7	17	3	na	11	3	14	814	na
Chicken, mushroom, canned, prepared w/water	1 cup (8 fl oz)	132	4	9	t	na	9	2	10	942	na
Chicken noodle, canned, prepared w/water	1 cup	75	4	9	1	na	2	1	7	1,106	na
Chicken noodle, chunky, ready-to-serve	1 serving	114	8	14	na	na	3	1	24	875	na
Chicken noodle, dehydrated, prepared w/water	1 cup	43	2	7	t	na	1	t	8	433	na
Chicken noodle with celery and onions, ready-to-serve	1 serving	95	6	9	na	na	3	1	21	985	na
Chicken vegetable, canned, prepared w/water	1 cup	75	4	9	1	na	3	1	10	945	na
Chicken vegetable, chunky, reduced-fat, reduced-sodium, ready-to-serve	1 serving	96	6	15	na	na	1	t	10	461	na

Food	Serving	Cal	Prot (g)	Carb (g)	Fiber (g)	Sugars (g)	Total Fat (g)	Sat/Trans Fat (g)	Chol (g)	Sod (mg)	GI
Chicken vegetable, dehydrated, prepared w/water	1 cup	50	3	8	na	na	1	t	3	808	na
Chicken w/dumplings, canned, prepared w/water	1 cup (8 fl oz)	96	6	6	.5	na	6	1	34	860	na
Chicken with rice, canned, prepared w/water	1 cup	60	4	7	1	na	2	t	7	815	na
Clam chowder, Manhattan style, canned, prepared w/water	1 cup	78	2	12	1.5	na	2	t	2	578	na
Clam chowder, Manhattan style, chunky, ready-to-serve	1 cup	134	7	19	3	na	3	2	14	1,001	na
Clam chowder, New England, canned, prepared w/milk	1 cup (8 fl oz)	164	10	17	2	na	7	3	22	992	na
Clam chowder, New England style, canned, prepared w/water	1 cup	95	5	12	1.5	na	3	t	5	915	na
Consomme, canned, prepared w/water	1 cup	29	5	2	0	na	2	0	0	636	na
Crab soup, ready-to-serve	1 cup	76	5	10	1	na	2	t/0	10	1,235	na

Food	Serving	Cal	Prot (g)	Carb (g)	Fiber (g)	Sugars (g)	Total Fat (g)	Sat/Trans Fat (g)	Chol (g)	Sod (mg)	GI
Cream of asparagus, canned, prepared w/milk	1 cup (8 fl oz)	161	6	16	1	na	8	3/na	22	1,042	na
Cream of asparagus, dehydrated, prepared w/water	1 cup	58	2	9	na	na	2	t/0	0	801	na
Cream of celery, canned, prepared w/milk	1 cup (8 fl oz)	164	6	15	1	na	10	4/na	32	1,009	na
Cream of celery, dehydrated, prepared w/water	1 cup	64	3	10	na	na	2	t/0	0	838	na
Cream of chicken, canned, prepared w/milk	1 cup (8 fl oz)	191	7	15	t	9	11	5/na	27	1,047	na
Cream of mushroom, canned, prepared w/milk	1 cup (8 fl oz)	203	6	15	.5	1.5	14	5/na	20	918	na
Cream of mushroom, canned, prepared w/water	1 cup (8 fl oz)	129	2	9	.5	na	9	2/0	2	881	na
Cream of onion, canned, prepared w/milk	1 cup (8 fl oz)	186	7	18	1	na	9	4/na	32	1,004	na
Cream of onion, canned, prepared w/water	1 cup (8 fl oz)	107	3	13	1	na	5	1/0	15	927	na

Food	Serving	Cal	Prot (g)	Carb (g)	Fiber (g)	Sugars (g)	Total Fat (g)	Sat/Trans Fat (g)	Chol (g)	Sod (mg)	GI
Cream of potato, canned, prepared w/milk	1 cup (8 fl oz)	149	6	17	.5	na	6	4/na	22	1,061	na
Cream of potato, canned, prepared w/water	1 cup	73	2	11	.5	na	2	1/0	5	1,000	na
Cream of shrimp, canned, prepared w/milk	1 cup (8 fl oz)	164	7	14	t	8	9	6/na	35	1,037	na
Cream of shrimp, canned, prepared w/water	1 cup (8 fl oz)	90	3	8	t	.5	5	3/0	17	976	na
Cream of vegetable, dehydrated, prepared w/water	1 cup (8 fl oz)	107	2	12	.5	.5	6	1/0	0	1,170	na
Gazpacho, ready-to-serve	1 cup	46	7	4	.5	1.5	t	t/0	0	739	na
Leek soup, dehydrated, prepared w/water	1 cup	71	2	11	3	na	2	1/0	3	965	na
Lentil soup, ready-to-serve	1 cup	126	8	20	6	na	1.5	t/0	0	443	44
Minestrone, chunky, ready-to-serve	1 cup	127	5	21	6	5	3	1/0	5	864	39
Minestrone, canned, prepared w/water	1 cup	82	4	11	1	na	2.5	t/0	2	911	39

241

Food	Serving	Cal	Prot (g)	Carb (g)	Fiber (g)	Sugars (g)	Total Fat (g)	Sat/Trans Fat (g)	Chol (g)	Sod (mg)	GI
Minestrone, dehydrated, prepared w/water	1 cup	79	4	12	na	na	2	1/0	3	1,026	39
Mushroom, dehydrated, prepared w/water	1 packet	74	2	9	1	.5	4	1/0	0	782	na
Mushroom barley, canned, prepared w/water	1 cup	73	2	12	1	na	2	t/0	0	891	na
Mushroom with beef stock, canned, prepared w/water	1 cup	85	3	9	1	na	4	1.5/0	7	969	na
Onion, canned, prepared w/water	1 cup	58	4	8	1	3	2	t/0	0	1,053	na
Onion, dehydrated, prepared w/water	1 cup	27	1	5	1	2	t	t/0	0	849	na
Oyster stew, canned, prepared w/milk	1 cup (8 fl oz)	135	6	10	0	na	8	5/na	32	1,041	na
Oyster stew, canned, prepared w/water	1 cup	58	2	4	na	na	4	2.5/0	14	981	na
Pea, green, canned, prepared w/milk	1 cup (8 fl oz)	239	13	32	3	na	7	4/na	18	970	66

242

Food	Serving	Cal	Prot (g)	Carb (g)	Fiber (g)	Sugars (g)	Total Fat (g)	Sat/Trans Fat (g)	Chol (g)	Sod (mg)	GI
Pea soup, canned, prepared w/water	1 cup	165	9	27	3	8	3	1/na	0	918	66
Pea soup, dehydrated, prepared w/water	1 cup	101	6	17	2	na	1	t/0	2	927	66
Potato ham chowder, chunky, ready-to-serve	1 serving	192	6	13	1	na	12	4/na	22	874	na
Sirloin burger w/vegetables, ready-to-serve	1 serving	185	10	16	6	na	9	3/na	26	866	na
Split pea, ready-to-serve	1 cup	180	10	30	5	5	2	1/0	5	420	60
Split pea w/ham, chunky, ready-to-serve	1 cup (8 fl oz)	185	11	27	4	na	4	2/0	7	965	60
Split pea w/ham, canned, prepared w/water	1 cup (8 fl oz)	190	10	28	2	na	4	2/0	8	1,007	60
Split pea w/ham, chunky, reduced-fat, reduced-sodium, ready-to-serve	1 serving	185	13	27	na	na	3	1/0	15	833	60
Tomato, canned, prepared w/milk	1 cup (8 fl oz)	161	6	22	3	na	6	3/0	17	744	38

Food	Serving	Cal	Prot (g)	Carb (g)	Fiber (g)	Sugars (g)	Total Fat (g)	Sat/Trans Fat (g)	Chol (g)	Sod (mg)	GI
Tomato, canned, prepared w/ water	1 cup	85	2	17	.5	9	2	t/0	0	695	38
Tomato, dehydrated, prepared w/ water	1 packet	78	2	15	t	10	2	1/0	0	708	38
Tomato beef w/noodle, canned, prepared w/water	1 cup (8 fl oz)	139	4	21	1	1	4	2/0	5	917	na
Tomato bisque, canned, prepared w/milk	1 cup (8 fl oz)	198	6	29	.5	na	7	3/na	23	1,109	na
Tomato bisque, canned, prepared w/ water	1 cup	124	2	24	.5	na	2.5	.5/0	5	1,047	na
Tomato rice, canned, prepared w/ water	1 cup	119	2	22	1.5	7	3	.5/0	2	815	na
Tomato vegetable, dehydrated, prepared w/water	1 packet	42	1	8	t	2.5	1	t/0	0	856	na
Turkey, chunky, ready-to-serve	1 cup	135	10	14	na	na	4	1/0	9	923	na
Turkey noodle, canned, prepared w/water	1 cup	68	4	9	1	na	2	t/0	5	815	na

244

Food	Serving	Cal	Prot (g)	Carb (g)	Fiber (g)	Sugars (g)	Total Fat (g)	Sat/Trans Fat (g)	Chol (g)	Sod (mg)	GI
Turkey vegetable, canned, prepared w/water	1 cup	72	3	9	.5	na	3	1/0	2	906	na
Vegetable, chunky, ready-to-serve	1 cup	122	3.5	19	1	na	4	.5/0	0	1,010	na
Vegetable beef, canned, prepared w/water	1 cup	78	6	10	.5	1	2	1/0	5	791	na
Vegetable beef, dehydrated, prepared w/water	1 cup	53	3	8	.5	1	1	.5/0	0	1,002	na
Vegetable beef, microwaveable, ready-to-serve	1 serving	128	18	10	4	na	2	1/0	9	1,098	na
Vegetable with beef broth, canned, prepared w/water	1 cup	82	3	13	.5	3	2	t/0	2	810	na
Vegetarian vegetable, canned, prepared w/water	1 cup	72	2	12	.5	3.5	2	t/0	0	822	na
SOY PRODUCTS											
Black bean burger (Worthington Foods, Morningstar Farms)	1 patty	150	16	19	4	2	6	1/0	2	587	na
Soybeans, boiled, w/salt	½ cup	149	14	9	5	2.5	8	2/0	0	204	18
Soybeans, boiled, w/o salt	½ cup	149	14	9	5	2.5	8	2/0	0	1	18

Food	Serving	Cal	Prot (g)	Carb (g)	Fiber (g)	Sugars (g)	Total Fat (g)	Sat/Trans Fat (g)	Chol (g)	Sod (mg)	GI
Soybeans, dry roasted, w/o salt	2 tbsp	101	9	7	2	na	5	1/0	0	0	na
Soy burger	1 patty	110	12	9	3	1	6	1/0	na	na	na
Soy cheese, Swiss	2 slices (0.7 oz)	120	11	1	na	na	8	na/na	na	na	na
Soy cheese, mozzarella	2 slices (1 oz)	120	15	2	na	na	6	na/na	na	na	na
Soy cheese, cheddar	2 slices (0.7 oz)	120	11	1	na	na	8	na/na	na	na	na
Soy cheese, American	2 slices (0.7 oz)	120	8	1	na	na	8	na/na	na	na	na
Soy milk, plain	1 cup	81	7	4	3	1	5	t/0	0	29	44
Soy pasta	1 serving (2 oz or ⅙ box)	200	14	34	1	2	2	1/0	0	85	47
Tempeh	½ cup	160	15	8	t	na	9	2/0	0	7	na
Tofu, silken, extra firm	1 slice	46	6	2	t	1	2	t/0	0	53	15
Tofu, silken, firm	1 slice	52	6	2	t	1	2	t/0	0	30	15
Tofu, silken, lite, extra firm	1 slice	32	6	1	0	na	t	t/0	0	82	15

246

Food	Serving	Cal	Prot (g)	Carb (g)	Fiber (g)	Sugars (g)	Total Fat (g)	Sat/Trans Fat (g)	Chol (g)	Sod (mg)	GI
Tofu, silken, soft	1 slice	46	4	2	na	1	2	t	0	4	15
Tofu, silken, lite, firm	1 slice	31	5	1	0	na	1	t	0	71	15
Vegetable burger	1 patty	138	18	7	6	na	4	1	0	411	na
SUGAR-FREE FOODS											
Candy, hard, sugar-free	1 candy	20	0	5	0	0	0	0/0	0	0	na
Gelatin dessert, sugar-free	½ cup	8	1	1	0	0	0	0/0	0	56	na
Gelatin, unflavored	1 envelope	23	6	0	0	0	0	0/0	0	14	na
Jelly/preserves, low- or reduced-sugar	1 tbsp	24	0	6	0	4.5	0	0/0	0	0	na
Sugar substitute	1 packet	4	0	1	0	1	0	0/0	0	0	is
Syrup, sugar-free	2 tbsp	9	0	2	0	2	0	0/0	0	27	na
TOMATOES AND TOMATO PRODUCTS											
Tomatillos, medium, raw	1 tomatillo	11	t	2	1	1	t	t/0	0	0	na
Tomatillos, chopped, raw	1 cup	42	1	8	2.5	2.5	t	t/0	0	1	na

Food	Serving	Cal	Prot (g)	Carb (g)	Fiber (g)	Sugars (g)	Total Fat (g)	Sat/Trans Fat (g)	Chol (g)	Sod (mg)	GI
Tomatoes, crushed, canned	½ cup	39	2	9	2	na	t	t/0	0	161	na
Tomatoes, green, chopped, raw	1 cup	43	2	9	2	7	t	t/0	0	23	30
Tomatoes, green, slice, or wedge, raw	1 piece	5	t	1	t	1	t	t/0	0	3	30
Tomatoes, green, whole, raw	1 large tomato	44	2	9	2	7	t	t/0	0	24	30
Tomatoes, green, whole, raw	1 medium tomato	30	1	6	1	5	t	t/0	0	16	30
Tomatoes, green, whole, small, raw	1 small tomato	22	1	5	1	4	t	t/0	0	12	30
Tomatoes, orange, chopped, raw	1 cup	25	2	5	1	na	t	t/0	0	66	30
Tomatoes, orange, raw	1 tomato	18	1	4	1	na	t	t/0	0	47	30
Tomatoes, red, canned, stewed	½ cup	36	1	9	1	6	t	t/0	0	282	na
Tomatoes, red, canned, wedges in tomato juice	½ cup	34	1	8	na	3	t	t/0	0	283	na
Tomatoes, red, whole, canned, w/o salt	½ cup	23	1	5	1	3	t	t/0	0	12	na

Food	Serving	Cal	Prot (g)	Carb (g)	Fiber (g)	Sugars (g)	Total Fat (g)	Sat/Trans Fat (g)	Chol (g)	Sod (mg)	GI
Tomatoes, red, whole, canned, w/salt	½ cup	23	1	5	1	3	t	t/0	0	178	na
Tomatoes, red, canned, with green chiles	½ cup	18	1	4	na	3	t	t/0	0	483	na
Tomatoes, red, boiled, w/o salt	½ cup	32	1	7	1	3	t	t/0	0	13	na
Tomatoes, red, boiled, w/salt	½ cup	32	1	7	1	3	t	t/0	0	296	na
Tomatoes, red, slice (¼" thick)	1 slice	4	t	1	t	1	t	t/0	0	2	30
Tomatoes, red (¼ of a medium tomato, raw)	1 wedge	7	t	1	t	1	t	t/0	0	3	30
Tomatoes, red, whole, boiled, w/o salt	2 medium tomatoes	66	3	14	2.5	3	t	t/0	0	27	na
Tomatoes, red, whole, raw	1 large tomato	38	2	8	2	4	t	t/0	0	16	30
Tomatoes, red, whole, raw	1 medium tomato	26	1	6	1	4	t	t/0	0	11	30
Tomatoes, red, whole, raw	1 small tomato	19	1	4	1	4	t	t/0	0	8	30

Food	Serving	Cal	Prot (g)	Carb (g)	Fiber (g)	Sugars (g)	Total Fat (g)	Sat/Trans Fat (g)	Chol (g)	Sod (mg)	GI
Tomatoes, red, stewed	½ cup	40	1	7	1	na	t	t/0	0	230	na
Tomatoes, cherry, raw	1 cup	31	1	7	2	4	t	t/0	0	13	30
Tomatoes, cherry, raw	1 tomato	4	t	1	t	t	t	t/0	0	2	30
Tomatoes, red, chopped, raw	1 cup	38	2	8	2	5	t	t/0	0	16	30
Tomatoes, roma (Italian), raw	1 tomato	13	t	3	1	na	t	t/0	0	6	30
Tomatoes, sun-dried	½ cup	70	4	15	3	10	t	t/0	0	566	na
Tomatoes, sun-dried	1 piece	5	t	1	t	1	t	t/0	0	42	na
Tomatoes, sun-dried, packed in oil, drained	1 cup	234	6	26	0	6	15	2/0	na	293	na
Tomatoes, yellow, chopped, raw	1 cup	21	1	4	1	na	t	t/0	0	32	30
Tomatoes, yellow, whole, raw	1 tomato	32	2	6	1.5	na	t	t/0	0	49	30
Tomato paste, w/o salt	¼ cup	54	2	10	2.5	na	t	t/0	0	57	na
Tomato paste, w/salt	¼ cup	54	3	12	3	8	t	t/0	0	517	na
Tomato puree, w/o salt	½ cup	54	3	12	2.5	8	t	t/0	0	64	na
Tomato puree, w/salt	½ cup	48	2	11	2.5	6	t	t/0	0	499	na

Food	Serving	Cal	Prot (g)	Carb (g)	Fiber (g)	Sugars (g)	Total Fat (g)	Sat/Trans Fat (g)	Chol (g)	Sod (mg)	GI
Tomato sauce, canned	½ cup	37	2	9	2	5	t	t/0	0	741	35–45
Tomato sauce, canned, Spanish style	½ cup	40	2	9	2	na	t	t/0	0	576	35–45
Tomato sauce, canned, w/ mushrooms	½ cup	43	2	10	2	6	t	t/0	0	554	35–45
Tomato sauce, canned, w/onions	½ cup	51	2	12	2	na	t	t/0	0	675	35–45
Tomato sauce, canned, w/onions, green peppers, and celery	½ cup	51	1	11	2	9	t	t/0	0	683	35–45
Tomato sauce, canned, w/tomato tidbits	½ cup	39	2	9	2	na	t	t/0	0	18	35–45

Food	Serving	Cal	Prot (g)	Carb (g)	Fiber (g)	Sugars (g)	Total Fat (g)	Sat/Trans Fat (g)	Chol (g)	Sod (mg)
TURKEY										
Back meat, w/o skin, roasted	4 oz	192	32	0	0	0	6	2/0	107	82
Boneless, roast, light and dark meat	4 oz	175	24	3	0	na	7	2/0	60	768
Breast meat, w/o skin, roasted	4 oz	153	34	0	0	0	1	t/0	94	59
Breast, meat and skin, roasted	4 oz	141	25	0	0	0	4	1/0	47	445
Canned, meat only, with broth	4 oz	184	27	0	0	0	8	2/0	75	528
Dark meat, roasted	4 oz	183	32	0	0	0	5	2/0	127	89
Dark meat, meat and skin, roasted	1 cup	309	38.5	0	0	0	16	5/0	125	106
Ground turkey	1 patty, 4 oz	193	22	0	0	0	11	3/0	84	88
Leg meat, w/o skin, roasted	4 oz	180	33	0	0	0	4	1/0	134	92
Light meat, all classes, roasted	4 oz	177	34	0	0	0	4	1/0	78	72
Light meat, meat and skin, roasted	1 cup	276	40	0	0	0	12	3/0	106	88
Meat, all classes, roasted	4 oz	192	33	0	0	0	6	2/0	86	79
Neck meat, w/o skin, cooked	4 oz	203	30	0	0	0	8	3/0	138	63

252

Food	Serving	Cal	Prot (g)	Carb (g)	Fiber (g)	Sugars (g)	Total Fat (g)	Sat/Trans Fat (g)	Chol (g)	Sod (mg)
Turkey, canned	1 can (5 oz)	204	30	0	0	0	9	2.5/0	83	584
Turkey ham	4 oz	134	18	4	0	1	5	1/0	73	1,031
Turkey leg, meat and skin, roasted	½ leg	568	76	0	0	0	27	8/0	232	210
Turkey wing, meat and skin, roasted	1 wing, bone removed	426	51	0	0	0	23	6/0	151	113
Turkey patties, battered, fried	1 patty	181	9	10	t	na	12	3/0	40	512
Turkey sticks, battered and fried	2 sticks	357	18	22	na	na	22	6/0	82	1,073
Turkey w/gravy, frozen	1 package	95	8	7	0	na	4	1/0	26	787
Wing, w/o skin and bone	1 wing	98	19	0	0	0	2	1/0	61	47
Young hen, dark meat, w/o skin, roasted	4 oz	217	32	0	0	0	9	3/0	90	85
Young hen, light meat, w/o skin, roasted	4 oz	182	34	0	0	0	4	1/0	77	68
Young hen, meat only, roasted	4 oz	198	33	0	0	0	6	2/0	82	76

Food	Serving	Cal	Prot (g)	Carb (g)	Fiber (g)	Sugars (g)	Total Fat (g)	Sat/Trans Fat (g)	Chol (g)	Sod (mg)
Young tom, dark meat, w/o skin, roasted	4 oz	209	32	0	0	0	8	3/0	99	93
Young tom, light meat, w/o skin, roasted	4 oz	174	34	0	0	0	3	1/0	78	77
Young tom, meat, w/o skin, roasted	4 oz	190	33	0	0	0	5	2/0	87	84
VEAL										
Breast, whole, lean only, boneless, braised	4 oz	247	34	0	0	0	11	4/0	131	77
Ground, broiled	4 oz	195	28	0	0	0	9	3/0	117	94
Leg, top round, lean only, braised	4 oz	230	42	0	0	0	6	2/0	153	76
Leg, top round, lean only, pan-fried	4 oz	207	38	0	0	0	5	1.5/0	121	87
Leg, top round, lean only, roasted	4 oz	170	32	0	0	0	4	1/0	117	77
Loin, braised	4 oz	156	23	0	0	0	6	2/0	86	58
Rib, braised	4 oz	247	39	0	0	0	9	3/0	163	112

Food	Serving	Cal	Prot (g)	Carb (g)	Fiber (g)	Sugars (g)	Total Fat (g)	Sat/Trans Fat (g)	Chol (g)	Sod (mg)
Rib, roasted	4 oz	201	29	0	0	0	8	2/0	130	110
Shank, lean only, braised	4 oz	201	37	0	0	0	5	1/0	143	107
Shoulder, arm, braised	4 oz	228	40	0	0	0	6	2/0	176	102
Shoulder, arm, lean only, roasted	4 oz	186	30	0	0	0	7	3/0	124	103
Shoulder, blade, lean only, braised	4 oz	224	37	0	0	0	7	2/0	179	114
Shoulder, blade, lean only, roasted	4 oz	194	29	0	0	0	8	3/0	135	116
Shoulder, whole (arm and shoulder), lean only, braised	4 oz	226	38	0	0	0	7	2/0	147	110
Shoulder, whole (arm and shoulder), lean only, roasted	4 oz	193	29	0	0	0	8	3/0	129	110
Sirloin, lean only, braised	4 oz	231	38	0	0	0	7	2/0	128	92
Sirloin, lean only, roasted	4 oz	190	30	0	0	0	7	3/0	118	96

Food	Serving	Cal	Prot (g)	Carb (g)	Fiber (g)	Sugars (g)	Total Fat (g)	Sat/Trans Fat (g)	Chol (g)	Sod (mg)	GI
VEGETABLES											
Acorn squash, cubes, baked, w/o salt	½ cup	57	1	15	4.5	na	t	t/0	0	4	75
Acorn squash, mashed, baked, w/o salt	½ cup	42	1	11	3	na	t	t/0	0	4	75
Alfalfa sprouts, raw	1 cup	10	1	1	1	na	t	t/0	0	2	na
Artichoke, hearts, canned in water	½ cup	37	3	6	4	0	0	0/0	0	891	15
Artichoke, hearts, boiled, drained, w/salt	½ cup	42	3	9	5	na	t	t/0	0	278	15
Artichoke, hearts, boiled, drained, w/o salt	½ cup	42	3	9	5	na	t	t/0	0	80	15
Artichoke, whole, globe or French boiled, drained w/salt	1 medium	60	4	13	7	na	t	t/0	0	397	15
Arugula, raw, chopped	1 cup	6	t	1	t	t	t	t/0	0	6	na
Asparagus, canned, drained	½ cup	23	3	3	2	1	t	t/0	0	347	15
Asparagus, from fresh, cuts and tips, cooked, w/ salt	½ cup	22	2	4	2	.5	t	t/0	0	216	15

Food	Serving	Cal	Prot (g)	Carb (g)	Fiber (g)	Sugars (g)	Total Fat (g)	Sat/Trans Fat (g)	Chol (g)	Sod (mg)	GI
Asparagus, from fresh, cuts and tips, cooked, w/o salt	½ cup	22	2	4	1	.5	t	t/0	0	10	15
Asparagus, from fresh, spears, boiled and drained, w/salt	6 spears	22	2	4	2	1	t	t/0	0	216	15
Asparagus, from fresh, spears, boiled and drained, w/o salt	6 spears	22	2	4	1	1	t	t/0	0	10	15
Asparagus, from frozen, cuts and tips, boiled, drained, w/salt	½ cup	25	3	4	1	t	t	t/0	0	216	15
Asparagus, from frozen, spears, boiled, drained, w/salt	6 spears	25	3	4	1	t	t	t/0	0	216	15
Bamboo shoots, canned, drained slices, w/salt	½ cup	7	1	1	1	1	t	t/0	0	144	20
Bamboo shoots, canned, drained slices, w/o salt	½ cup	12	1	2	1	1	t	t/0	0	5	20
Bamboo shoots, raw, pieces	1 cup	41	4	8	3	2	t	t/0	0	6	20
Beans, snap, green, canned, w/salt	½ cup	14	1	3	1	t	t	t/0	0	177	15
Beans, snap, green, canned, w/o salt	½ cup	14	1	3	1	t	t	t/0	0	1	15

Food	Serving	Cal	Prot (g)	Carb (g)	Fiber (g)	Sugars (g)	Total Fat (g)	Sat/Trans Fat (g)	Chol (g)	Sod (mg)	GI
Beans, snap, green, from fresh, boiled, w/salt	½ cup	22	1	5	2	1	t	t/0	0	149	15
Beans, snap, green, from fresh, boiled, w/o salt	½ cup	22	1	5	2	1	t	t/0	0	2	15
Beans, snap, green, from frozen, boiled, w/salt	½ cup	19	1	4	2	1	t	t/0	0	165	15
Beans, snap, green, from frozen, boiled, w/o salt	½ cup	19	1	4	2	1	t	t/0	0	6	15
Beans, snap, green, raw	1 cup	34	2	8	4	1.5	t	t/0	0	7	15
Beans, snap, yellow, canned, w/salt	½ cup	14	1	3	1	t	t	t/0	0	169	15
Beans, snap, yellow, canned, w/o salt	½ cup	14	1	3	1	t	t	t/0	0	1	15
Beans, snap, yellow, from fresh, boiled, w/salt	½ cup	22	1	5	2	1	t	t/0	0	149	15
Beans, snap, yellow, from fresh, boiled, w/o salt	½ cup	22	1	5	2	1	t	t/0	0	2	15

Food	Serving	Cal	Prot (g)	Carb (g)	Fiber (g)	Sugars (g)	Total Fat (g)	Sat/Trans Fat (g)	Chol (g)	Sod (mg)	GI
Beans, snap, yellow, from frozen, boiled, w/salt	½ cup	19	1	4	2	1	t	t/0	0	165	15
Beans, snap, yellow, from frozen, boiled, w/o salt	½ cup	19	1	4	2	1	t	t/0	0	6	15
Beans, snap, yellow, raw	1 cup	34	2	8	4	1.5	t	t/0	0	7	15
Beets, raw	1 cup	58	2	13	4	9	t	t/0	0	106	30
Beets, raw (2" dia.)	2 beets	71	3	16	5	5.5	t	t/0	0	128	30
Beets, canned, diced, drained	½ cup	24	1	6	1	4	t	t/0	0	152	65
Beets, canned, shredded, drained	½ cup	30	1	7	2	5.5	t	t/0	0	189	65
Beets, canned, sliced, drained	½ cup	26	1	6	1	6	t	t/0	0	165	65
Beets, canned, whole, drained	½ cup	25	1	6	1	6	t	t/0	0	158	65
Beets, canned, drained	2 beets	15	t	3	1	8	t	t/0	0	93	65
Beets, from fresh, sliced, boiled, drained	½ cup	37	1	8	2	4	t	t/0	0	65	65
Beets, canned, pickled, sliced	½ cup	74	1	18	3	4	t	t/0	0	300	65

Food	Serving	Cal	Prot (g)	Carb (g)	Fiber (g)	Sugars (g)	Total Fat (g)	Sat/Trans Fat (g)	Chol (g)	Sod (mg)	GI
Beets, whole, from fresh, cooked	2 beets	44	2	10	2	8	t	t/0	0	77	65
Beets, Harvard, canned, sliced	½ cup	90	1	22	3	na	t	t/0	0	199	65
Beet greens, boiled, drained, w/salt	½ cup	19	2	4	2	t	t	t/0	0	343	na
Beet greens, boiled, drained, w/o salt	½ cup	19	2	4	2	t	t	t/0	0	174	na
Beet greens, raw, chopped	1 cup	7	1	2	1	t	t	t/0	0	76	na
Breadfruit, cooked	½ cup	113	1	30	5	12	t	t/0	0	2	15
Broccoli, Chinese, cooked	½ cup	10	t	2	1	t	t	t/0	0	3	15
Broccoli, boiled, drained, w/o salt	1 large stalk (11"–12" long)	78	8	14	8	1	1	t/0	0	73	15
Broccoli, boiled, drained, w/o salt	1 medium stalk (7½"–8" long)	50	5	9	5	1	1	t/0	0	47	15

Food	Serving	Cal	Prot (g)	Carb (g)	Fiber (g)	Sugars (g)	Total Fat (g)	Sat/Trans Fat (g)	Chol (g)	Sod (mg)	GI
Broccoli, boiled, drained, w/o salt	1 small stalk (5" long)	39	4	7	4	1	t	t/0	0	36	15
Broccoli, chopped, boiled, drained, w/o salt	½ cup	22	2	4	2	1	t	t/0	0	20	15
Broccoli flowerets, raw	1 cup	20	2	4	na	na	t	t/0	0	19	15
Broccoli, frozen, chopped, boiled, drained, w/o salt	½ cup	26	3	5	3	1	t	t/0	0	22	15
Broccoli, frozen, spears, boiled, drained, w/o salt	½ cup	26	3	5	3	1	t	t/0	0	22	15
Broccoli, raw, chopped	1 cup	25	3	5	3	1.5	t	t/0	0	24	15
Broccoli, raw, spears	2 spears	17	2	3	2	1	t	t/0	0	17	15
Broccoli, raw, stalk	1 stalk	42	5	8	4.5	t	t	t/0	0	41	15
Brussels sprouts, boiled, drained, w/o salt	6 sprouts	49	3	11	3	.5	t	t/0	0	26	15
Brussels sprouts, boiled, drained, w/o salt	½ cup	30	2	7	2	.5	t	t/0	0	16	15

Food	Serving	Cal	Prot (g)	Carb (g)	Fiber (g)	Sugars (g)	Total Fat (g)	Sat/Trans Fat (g)	Chol (g)	Sod (mg)	GI
Brussels sprouts, frozen, boiled, drained, w/o salt	½ cup	33	3	6	3	.5	t	t/0	0	18	15
Brussels sprouts, raw	1 cup	38	3	8	3	2	t	t/0	0	22	15
Brussels sprouts, raw	6 sprouts	49	4	10	4	2.5	t	t/0	0	29	15
Butternut squash, cubes, baked, w/o salt	½ cup	41	1	11	na	2	t	t/0	0	4	75
Butternut squash, frozen, boiled, w/o salt	½ cup	47	1	12	na	2	t	t/0	0	2	75
Cabbage, Chinese (pak-choi), shredded, boiled, drained, w/o salt	½ cup	10	1	2	1	t	t	t/0	0	29	15
Cabbage, Chinese (pak-choi), shredded, raw	1 cup	9	1	2	1	t	t	t/0	0	46	15
Cabbage, Chinese (pe-tsai), shredded, boiled, drained, w/o salt	½ cup	8	1	1	1	na	t	t/0	0	5	15
Cabbage, Chinese (pe-tsai), shredded, raw	1 cup	12	1	2	2	na	t	t/0	0	7	15

262

Food	Serving	Cal	Prot (g)	Carb (g)	Fiber (g)	Sugars (g)	Total Fat (g)	Sat/Trans Fat (g)	Chol (g)	Sod (mg)	GI
Cabbage, raw, chopped	1 cup	22	1	5	2	3	t	t/0	0	16	15
Cabbage, raw, shredded	1 cup	18	1	4	2	2	t	t/0	0	13	15
Cabbage, shredded, boiled, drained, w/o salt	½ cup	17	1	3	2	1	t	t/0	0	6	15
Cabbage, napa, cooked	½ cup	7	1	1	na	na	t	t/0	0	6	15
Cabbage, red, shredded, boiled, drained, w/o salt	½ cup	16	1	3	1.5	2.5	t	t/0	0	6	15
Cabbage, red, raw, chopped	1 cup	24	1	5	5.5	3	t	t/0	0	10	15
Cabbage, red, raw, shredded	1 cup	19	1	4	1	3	t	t/0	0	8	15
Cabbage, savoy, raw, shredded	1 cup	19	1	4	2	1.5	t	t/0	0	20	15
Cabbage, savoy, shredded, boiled, drained, w/o salt	½ cup	17	1	4	2	na	t	t/0	0	133	15
Carrots, baby, large, raw	6	34	1	7	2	1	t	t/0	0	31	30
Carrots, baby, medium, raw	6	23	t	5	1	3	t	t/0	0	21	na
Carrots, canned, mashed, w/o salt	½ cup	29	1	6	2	3	t	t/0	0	48	85

263

Food	Serving	Cal	Prot (g)	Carb (g)	Fiber (g)	Sugars (g)	Total Fat (g)	Sat/Trans Fat (g)	Chol (g)	Sod (mg)	GI
Carrots, canned, sliced, w/o salt	½ cup	18	t	4	1	2	t	t/0	0	31	85
Carrots, raw, chopped	1 cup	55	1	13	4	6	t	t/0	0	45	47
Carrots, raw, grated	1 cup	47	1	11	3	5	t	t/0	0	39	47
Carrots, raw, sliced	1 cup	52	1	12	4	6	t	t/0	0	43	47
Carrots, sliced, boiled, drained, w/o salt	½ cup	35	1	8	3	1.5	t	t/0	0	51	85
Carrots, frozen, sliced, boiled, w/o salt	½ cup	26	1	6	3	1.5	t	t/0	0	43	85
Cauliflower, raw	1 cup	25	2	5	2.5	2	t	t/0	0	30	15
Cauliflower, raw, flowerets	6	20	2	4	2	t	t	t/0	0	23	15
Cauliflower, boiled, drained, w/o salt	½ cup	14	1	3	2	t	t	t/0	0	9	15
Cauliflower, flowerets, boiled, drained, w/o salt	6 pieces	25	2	4	3	t	t	t/0	0	16	15
Cauliflower, frozen, boiled, drained, w/o salt	½ cup	17	1	3	2	t	t	t/0	0	16	15

Food	Serving	Cal	Prot (g)	Carb (g)	Fiber (g)	Sugars (g)	Total Fat (g)	Sat/Trans Fat (g)	Chol (g)	Sod (mg)	GI
Cauliflower, green, cooked, w/o salt	¼ head	29	3	6	3	t	t	t/0	0	21	15
Cauliflower, green, raw	1 cup	20	2	4	2	2	t	t/0	0	15	15
Cauliflower, green, flowerets	6	47	4	9	5	2	t	t/0	0	35	15
Celery, diced, boiled, drained, w/o salt	½ cup	14	t	3	1	t	t	t/0	0	68	15
Celery, diced, raw	1 cup	19	1	4	2	t	t	t/0	0	104	15
Celery, strips, raw	1 cup	20	1	5	2	t	t	t/0	0	108	15
Chard, Swiss, chopped, boiled, drained, w/o salt	½ cup	18	2	4	2	t	t	t/0	0	157	na
Chard, Swiss, raw	1 cup	7	1	1	1	t	t	t/0	0	77	na
Chayote, chopped, boiled, drained, w/o salt	½ cup	19	t	4	2	t	t	t/0	0	1	50
Chayote, chopped, raw	1 cup	25	1	6	2	2.4	t	t/0	0	3	50
Collards, chopped, boiled, drained, w/o salt	½ cup	25	2	5	3	t	t	t/0	0	9	na

Food	Serving	Cal	Prot (g)	Carb (g)	Fiber (g)	Sugars (g)	Total Fat (g)	Sat/Trans Fat (g)	Chol (g)	Sod (mg)	GI
Collards, chopped, frozen, boiled, drained, w/o salt	½ cup	31	3	6	2	t	t	t/0	0	43	na
Collards, chopped, raw	1 cup	11	1	2	1	t	t	t/0	0	7	na
Corn, canned, w/red and green peppers	½ cup	85	3	21	na	na	t	t/0	0	394	46
Corn, canned, white, sweet, whole kernel	½ cup	66	2	15	2	3	1	t/0	0	265	46
Corn, canned, white, sweet, whole kernel, w/o salt	½ cup	82	3	20	1	3	1	t/0	0	15	46
Corn, fresh, white, sweet, boiled, drained w/o salt	½ cup	89	3	21	2	3	1	t/0	0	14	46
Corn, frozen, white, sweet, boiled, drained, w/o salt	½ cup	66	2	16	2	3	t	t/0	0	4	46
Corn, white, sweet, on the cob	1 ear	59	2	14	2	na	t	t/0	0	151	46
Corn, canned, yellow, sweet	½ cup	66	2	15	2	4	1	t/0	0	175	46
Corn, fresh, yellow, sweet, boiled, drained, w/o salt	½ cup	88	3	20	3	2.5	1	t/0	0	14	46

Food	Serving	Cal	Prot (g)	Carb (g)	Fiber (g)	Sugars (g)	Total Fat (g)	Sat/Trans Fat (g)	Chol (g)	Sod (mg)	GI
Corn on the cob, fresh, yellow, sweet, boiled, drained, w/o salt	1 ear	83	3	19	2	2	1	t/0	0	13	46
Corn cut off the cob, frozen, yellow, sweet, boiled, drained, w/o salt	½ cup	66	2	16	2	2	t	t/0	0	4	46
Cucumber, peeled, raw, chopped	1 cup	16	1	3	1	2	t	t/0	0	3	15
Cucumber, peeled, raw, sliced	1 cup	14	1	3	1	2	t	t/0	0	2	15
Cucumber, peeled, raw, large (8¼" long)	1	34	2	7	2	4	t	t/0	0	6	15
Cucumber, peeled, raw, medium	1	24	1	5	1	3	t	t/0	0	4	15
Cucumber, peeled, raw, small (6⅜" long)	1	19	t	4	1	2	t	t/0	0	3	15
Cucumber, with peel, raw, slices	1 cup	14	1	3	1	2	t	t/0	0	2	15
Cucumber, with peel, raw, large (8¼" long)	1	39	2	8	2	6	t	t/0	0	6	15
Dandelion greens, chopped, boiled, drained, w/o salt	½ cup	17	1	3	1.5	t	t	t/0	0	23	na

267

Food	Serving	Cal	Prot (g)	Carb (g)	Fiber (g)	Sugars (g)	Total Fat (g)	Sat/Trans Fat (g)	Chol (g)	Sod (mg)	GI
Dandelion greens, raw, chopped	1 cup	25	1	5	2	t	t	t/0	0	42	na
Eggplant, cubes, boiled, drained, w/o salt	½ cup	14	t	3	1	1.5	t	t/0	0	1	15
Eggplant, raw, cubes	1 cup	21	1	5	2	1.5	t	t/0	0	2	15
Endive, raw, chopped	1 cup	9	t	2	2	t	t	t/0	0	11	na
Grape leaves, canned	4 leaves	11	t	2	na	na	t	0/0	0	456	na
Grape leaves, raw	1 cup	13	1	2	1.5	1	t	t/0	0	1	na
Jicama, raw, sliced	1 cup	46	1	11	6	2	t	t/0	0	5	na
Hubbard squash, baked, cubes, w/o salt	½ cup	51	3	11	3.5	3.5	t	t/0	0	8	na
Hubbard squash, boiled, mashed, w/o salt	½ cup	35	2	8	.5	3.5	t	t/0	0	6	75
Kale, chopped, boiled, drained, w/o salt	½ cup	18	1	4	1	t	t	t/0	0	15	na
Kale, frozen, chopped, boiled, drained, w/o salt	½ cup	20	2	3	1	t	t	t/0	0	10	na
Kale, raw, chopped	1 cup	34	2	7	1	t	t	t/0	0	29	na

268

Food	Serving	Cal	Prot (g)	Carb (g)	Fiber (g)	Sugars (g)	Total Fat (g)	Sat/Trans Fat (g)	Chol (g)	Sod (mg)	GI
Kale, scotch, chopped, boiled, drained, w/o salt	½ cup	18	1	4	1	t	t	t/0	0	29	na
Kale, scotch, raw, chopped	1 cup	28	2	6	1	t	t	t/0	0	47	na
Kohlrabi, sliced, boiled, drained, w/o salt	½ cup	24	1	6	1	2.5	t	t/0	0	17	na
Kohlrabi, raw	1 cup	36	2	8	5	2.5	t	t/0	0	27	na
Leeks (bulb and lower-leaf portion), boiled, drained, w/o salt	1 leek	38	1	10	1	na	t	t/0	0	12	15
Leeks, chopped (bulb and lower-leaf portion), boiled, drained, w/o salt	½ cup	16	t	4	t	na	t	t/0	0	5	15
Leeks, chopped, raw (bulb and lower-leaf portion)	1 cup	54	1	13	2	3.5	t	t/0	0	18	15
Leeks, raw (bulb and lower-leaf portion)	1 leek	54	1	13	2	3.5	t	t/0	0	18	15
Lettuce, shredded, raw, butterhead, boston, and bibb types	1 cup	7	1	1	1	t	t	t/0	0	3	15

269

Food	Serving	Cal	Prot (g)	Carb (g)	Fiber (g)	Sugars (g)	Total Fat (g)	Sat/Trans Fat (g)	Chol (g)	Sod (mg)	GI
Lettuce, shredded, raw, cos or romaine	1 cup	8	1	1	1	t	t	t/0	0	4	15
Lettuce, shredded, raw, iceberg	1 cup	7	1	1	1	t	t	t/0	0	5	15
Lettuce, shredded, raw, looseleaf	1 cup	10	1	2	1	t	t	t/0	0	5	15
Lettuce, shredded, raw, radicchio	1 cup	9	1	2	t	t	t	t/0	0	9	15
Mushrooms, raw, Crimini or Italian	6 pieces	18	2	4	.5	1	t	t/0	0	5	15
Mushrooms, canned, drained	½ cup	19	1	4	2	1.5	t	t/0	0	332	15
Mushrooms, boiled, drained, w/o salt	½ cup	21	2	4	2	1.5	t	t/0	0	2	15
Mushrooms, boiled, drained, w/o salt	6 pieces	19	2	4	2	1.5	t	t/0	0	1	15
Mushrooms, raw, enoki	6 pieces (large)	10	1	2	1	t	t	t/0	0	1	15
Mushrooms, raw, enoki	6 pieces (medium)	6	t	1	.5	t	t	t/0	0	1	15
Mushrooms, raw, slices or pieces	1 cup	18	2	3	1	t	t	t/0	0	3	15
Mushrooms, raw, whole	1 cup	24	3	4	1	t	t	t/0	0	4	15

Food	Serving	Cal	Prot (g)	Carb (g)	Fiber (g)	Sugars (g)	Total Fat (g)	Sat/Trans Fat (g)	Chol (g)	Sod (mg)	GI
Mushrooms, raw	6 pieces (large)	35	4	6	2	t	t	t/0	0	6	15
Mushrooms, raw	6 pieces (medium)	27	3	5	1	t	t	t/0	0	4	15
Mushrooms, raw portabella	4 slices	20	3	4	3	1	0	t/0	0	10	15
Mushrooms, cooked, pieces, shitake, w/o salt	½ cup	40	1	10	1.5	2.5	t	t/0	0	3	15
Mushrooms, cooked, whole, shitake, w/o salt	6 pieces	59	2	15	2	6	t	t/0	0	4	15
Mushrooms, dried, shitake	6 mush-rooms	67	2	17	3	t	t	t/0	0	3	15
Mushrooms, canned, straw, drained	½ cup	29	3	4	2	t	t	t/0	0	349	15
Okra, frozen, boiled, drained, w/o salt	½ cup	26	2	5	3	na	t	t/0	0	3	na
Okra, raw	1 cup	33	2	8	3	2	t	t/0	0	8	na
Okra, raw	6 pods	24	1	5	2	1.5	t	t/0	0	6	na

Food	Serving	Cal	Prot (g)	Carb (g)	Fiber (g)	Sugars (g)	Total Fat (g)	Sat/Trans Fat (g)	Chol (g)	Sod (mg)	GI
Okra, slices, boiled, drained, w/o salt	½ cup	26	1	6	2	2	t	t/0	0	4	na
Okra, whole, boiled, drained, w/o salt	6 pods	20	1	5	2	2	t	t/0	0	3	na
Onions, boiled, drained, w/o salt	½ cup	46	1	11	1.5	5	t	t/0	0	3	15
Onions, boiled, drained, w/o salt	1 large	56	2	13	2	6	t	t/0	0	4	15
Onions, boiled, drained, w/o salt	1 medium	41	1	10	1	4	t	t/0	0	3	15
Onions, boiled, drained, w/o salt	1 small	26	1	6	1	3	t	t/0	0	2	15
Onions, canned	½ cup	21	1	5	1	2.5	t	t/0	0	416	15
Onions, dehydrated flakes	¼ cup	49	1	12	1	5	t	t/0	0	3	15
Onions, frozen, chopped, boiled, drained, w/o salt	½ cup	29	1	7	2	5	t	t/0	0	13	15
Onions, raw, chopped	1 cup	61	2	14	3	3.5	t	t/0	0	5	15
Onions, raw, sliced	1 cup	44	1	10	2	2.5	t	t/0	0	3	15
Onions, raw, sliced (¼" thick)	1 slice	14	t	3	1	2	t	t/0	0	1	15
Onions, raw, sliced (⅛" thick)	1 slice	5	t	1	t	.5	t	t/0	0	0	15

272

Food	Serving	Cal	Prot (g)	Carb (g)	Fiber (g)	Sugars (g)	Total Fat (g)	Sat/Trans Fat (g)	Chol (g)	Sod (mg)	GI
Onions, raw, whole	1 large	57	2	13	3	6	t	t/0	0	5	15
Onions, raw, whole	1 medium	42	1	9	2	5	t	t/0	0	3	15
Onions, raw, whole	1 small	27	1	6	1	3	t	t/0	0	2	15
Onions, raw, chopped, spring or scallions (tops and bulbs)	1 cup	32	2	7	3	7	t	t/0	0	16	15
Onions, raw, whole, spring or scallions (tops and bulbs)	1 large	8	t	2	1	t	t	t/0	0	4	15
Onions, raw, whole, spring or scallions (tops and bulbs)	1 medium	5	t	1	t	t	t	t/0	0	2	15
Onions, raw, whole, spring or scallions (tops and bulbs)	1 small	2	t	t	t	t	t	t/0	0	1	15
Palm, hearts, canned	½ cup	20	2	3	2	na	t	t/0	0	311	na
Palm, hearts, canned	3 pieces	28	2.5	5	2	na	t	t/0	0	422	na
Parsley, freeze-dried	¼ cup	4	t	t	.5	na	t	t/0	0	5	na
Parsley, raw	1 cup	22	2	4	2	.5	t	t/0	0	34	na
Parsley, raw	6 sprigs	2	t	t	t	t	t	t/0	0	3	na

Food	Serving	Cal	Prot (g)	Carb (g)	Fiber (g)	Sugars (g)	Total Fat (g)	Sat/Trans Fat (g)	Chol (g)	Sod (mg)	GI
Parsnips, raw	1 cup	100	2	24	6.5	na	t	t/0	0	13	97
Parsnips, sliced, boiled, drained, w/o salt	½ cup	63	1	15	3	4	t	t/0	0	192	97
Parsnips, sliced, boiled, drained, w/o salt	½ cup	63	1	15	3	4	t	t/0	0	8	97
Peas and carrots, canned, w/o salt	½ cup	48	3	11	4	4	t	t/0	0	5	na
Peas and carrots, canned, w/salt	½ cup	48	3	11	3	4	t	t/0	0	332	na
Peas and carrots, frozen, boiled, drained, w/o salt	½ cup	38	3	8	2.5	1.5	t	t/0	0	243	na
Peas and carrots, frozen, boiled, drained, w/o salt	½ cup	38	3	8	2.5	1.5	t	t/0	0	54	na
Peas, edible-podded, fresh, boiled, drained, w/o salt	½ cup	34	3	6	2	3	t	t/0	0	3	48
Peas, edible-podded, frozen, boiled, drained, w/o salt	½ cup	42	3	7	2.5	3	t	t/0	0	4	48
Peas, green, canned, w/o salt	½ cup	59	4	11	3.5	3	t	t/0	0	2	48

Food	Serving	Cal	Prot (g)	Carb (g)	Fiber (g)	Sugars (g)	Total Fat (g)	Sat/Trans Fat (g)	Chol (g)	Sod (mg)	GI
Peas, green, fresh, boiled, drained, w/o salt	½ cup	67	4	13	5	4	t	t/0	0	2	48
Peas, green, frozen, boiled, drained, w/salt	½ cup	62	4	11	4	4	t	t/0	0	258	48
Peas, green, frozen, boiled, drained, w/o salt	½ cup	62	4	11	4	4	t	t/0	0	58	48
Peas, pigeon, fresh, boiled, w/o salt	½ cup	102	6	20	6	na	t	t/0	0	4	48
Peas and onions, canned	½ cup	31	2	5	1	na	t	t/0	0	265	na
Peas and onions, frozen, boiled, drained, w/salt	½ cup	41	2	8	2	3	t	t/0	0	33	na
Peas and onions, frozen, boiled, drained, w/o salt	½ cup	41	2	8	2	3	t	t/0	0	33	na
Peppers, chili, green, canned	½ cup	15	t	3	1	na	t	t/0	0	276	15
Peppers, hot chili, sun-dried	6 peppers	10	t	2	1	na	t	t/0	0	3	15
Peppers, hot chili, green, chopped, canned, pods	½ cup	14	t	3	1	na	t	t/0	0	798	15

Food	Serving	Cal	Prot (g)	Carb (g)	Fiber (g)	Sugars (g)	Total Fat (g)	Sat/Trans Fat (g)	Chol (g)	Sod (mg)	GI
Peppers, hot chili, green, whole, canned	1 pepper	15	t	4	1	2	t	t/0	0	856	15
Peppers, hot chili, green, chopped, raw	1 cup	60	3	14	2	8	t	t/0	0	11	15
Peppers, hot chili, green, whole, raw	1 pepper	18	1	4	1	8	t	t/0	0	3	15
Peppers, chili, red, chopped, canned	½ cup	14	t	3	1	4	t	t/0	0	798	15
Peppers, hot chili, red, whole, canned	1 pepper	15	t	4	1	2	t	t/0	0	856	15
Peppers, hot chili, red, chopped, raw	1 cup	60	3	14	2	4	t	t/0	0	11	15
Peppers, hot chili, red, whole, raw	1 pepper	18	1	4	1	2	t	t/0	0	3	15
Peppers, Hungarian, raw	1 pepper	8	t	2	na	na	t	t/0	0	0	15
Peppers, jalapeño, chopped, canned	½ cup	18	t	3	2	2	t	t/0	0	1,136	15
Peppers, jalapeño, sliced, canned	½ cup	14	t	2	1	2	t	t/0	0	869	15

Food	Serving	Cal	Prot (g)	Carb (g)	Fiber (g)	Sugars (g)	Total Fat (g)	Sat/Trans Fat (g)	Chol (g)	Sod (mg)	GI
Peppers, jalapeño, whole, canned	1 pepper	6	t	1	1	.5	t	t/0	0	368	15
Peppers, jalapeño, whole, raw	1 pepper	4	t	1	1	.5	t	t/0	0	0	15
Peppers, sweet, green, halves, canned	½ cup	13	t	3	1	na	t	t/0	0	958	15
Peppers, sweet, green, strips, boiled, drained, w/o salt	½ cup	19	t	5	1	3	t	t/0	0	1	15
Peppers, sweet, green, chopped, boiled, drained, w/o salt	½ cup	19	t	5	1	3	t	t/0	0	1	15
Peppers, sweet, green, chopped, raw	1 cup	40	1	10	3	2	t	t/0	0	3	15
Peppers, sweet, green, slices, raw	1 cup	25	1	6	2	2	t	t/0	0	2	15
Peppers, sweet, green, large, raw	1 pepper	44	1	11	3	4	t	t/0	0	3	15
Peppers, sweet, green, medium, raw	1 pepper	32	1	8	2	3	t	t/0	0	2	15
Peppers, sweet, green, small, raw	1 pepper	20	t	5	1	2	t	t/0	0	1	15
Peppers, sweet, green, rings, raw	6 rings	16	t	4	1	t	t	t/0	0	1	15
Peppers, sweet, green, strips, raw	6 strips	4	t	1	t	t	t	t/0	0	0	15

Food	Serving	Cal	Prot (g)	Carb (g)	Fiber (g)	Sugars (g)	Total Fat (g)	Sat/Trans Fat (g)	Chol (g)	Sod (mg)	GI
Peppers, sweet, red, strips, boiled, drained, w/o salt	½ cup	19	t	5	1	na	t	t/0	0	1	15
Peppers, sweet, red, chopped, boiled, drained, w/o salt	½ cup	19	t	5	1	4	t	t/0	0	1	15
Peppers, sweet, red, chopped, raw	1 cup	40	1	10	3	3	t	t/0	0	3	15
Peppers, sweet, red, slices, raw	1 cup	25	1	6	2	na	t	t/0	0	2	15
Peppers, sweet, red, large, raw	1 pepper	44	1	11	3	7	t	t/0	0	3	15
Peppers, sweet, red, medium, raw	1 pepper	32	1	8	2	5	t	t/0	0	2	15
Peppers, sweet, red, small, raw	1 pepper	20	t	5	1.5	3	t	t/0	0	1	15
Peppers, sweet, yellow, large, raw	1 pepper	50	2	12	2	na	t	t/0	0	4	15
Peppers, sweet, yellow, strips, raw	6 strips	8	t	2	t	t	t	t/0	0	1	15
Potato, baked with skin, w/salt	1 medium	161	4	37	4	2	t	t/0	0	422	85
Potato, baked with skin, w/o salt	1 medium	161	4	37	4	2	t	t/0	0	17	85
Potato, boiled w/o skin, w/o salt	1 medium	144	3	33	3	1	t	t/0	0	8	85
Potatoes, canned, drained	½ cup	54	1	12	2	na	t	t/0	0	197	63

278

Food	Serving	Cal	Prot (g)	Carb (g)	Fiber (g)	Sugars (g)	Total Fat (g)	Sat/Trans Fat (g)	Chol (g)	Sod (mg)	GI
Potatoes, microwaved with skin, w/salt	1 medium	156	3	36	2.5	na	t	t/0	0	379	85
Potatoes, red, baked w/flesh and skin	1 medium	154	4	34	3	2.5	t	t/0	0	14	85
Potatoes, Russet, baked w/flesh and skin	1 medium	168	5	37	4	2	t	t/0	0	14	94
Pumpkin, canned, w/o salt	½ cup	42	1	10	4	4	t	t/0	0	6	na
Pumpkin, canned, w/o salt	½ cup	42	1	10	4	4	t	t/0	0	6	75
Pumpkin, boiled, mashed, w/salt	½ cup	25	1	6	1	1	t	t/0	0	162	na
Pumpkin, boiled, mashed, w/o salt	½ cup	25	1	6	1	1	t	t/0	0	1	75
Radishes, oriental, sliced, boiled, drained, w/o salt	½ cup	12	t	3	1	1	t	t/0	0	10	15
Radishes, oriental, whole, raw	1 radish	61	2	14	5	8.5	t	t/0	0	71	15
Radishes, slices, raw	1 cup	23	1	4	2	2	t	t/0	0	28	15
Radish, large, raw	1 radish	2	t	t	t	t	t	t/0	0	2	15
Radish, medium, raw	1 radish	1	t	t	t	t	t	t/0	0	1	15

Food	Serving	Cal	Prot (g)	Carb (g)	Fiber (g)	Sugars (g)	Total Fat (g)	Sat/Trans Fat (g)	Chol (g)	Sod (mg)	GI
Radishes, white icicle, slices, raw	1 cup	14	1	3	1	na	t	t/0	0	16	15
Radishes, white icicle, whole, raw	1 radish	2	t	t	t	na	t	t/0	0	3	15
Rutabagas, cubes, boiled, drained, w/o salt	½ cup	33	1	7	1.5	7	t	t/0	0	17	na
Rutabagas, mashed, boiled, drained, w/o salt	½ cup	47	2	11	2	7	t	t/0	0	24	na
Sauerkraut, canned	½ cup	13	t	3	2	2.5	t	t/0	0	469	15
Seaweed, kelp, raw	2 tbsp	34	1	8	1	t	t	t/0	0	186	na
Shallots, chopped, raw	1 tbsp	7	t	2	na	na	t	t/0	0	1	15
Spinach, canned, w/o salt	½ cup	22	2	3	3	t	t	t/0	0	88	15
Spinach, boiled, drained, w/o salt	½ cup	21	3	3	2	t	t	t/0	0	63	15
Spinach, frozen, chopped or leaf, boiled, drained, w/o salt	½ cup	27	3	5	3	t	t	t/0	0	82	15
Spinach, raw	1 cup	7	1	1	1	t	t	t/0	0	24	15
Split peas, boiled, w salt	½ cup	116	8	21	8	3	t	t/0	0	2	32
Split peas, boiled, w/o salt	½ cup	116	8	21	8	3	t	t/0	0	2	32
Sprouts, alfalfa, raw	1 cup	10	1	1	1	t	t	t/0	0	2	15

280

Food	Serving	Cal	Prot (g)	Carb (g)	Fiber (g)	Sugars (g)	Total Fat (g)	Sat/Trans Fat (g)	Chol (g)	Sod (mg)	GI
Sprouts, Mung, boiled, drained	½ cup	13	1	2.5	na	1.5	t	t/0	0	na	15
Sprouts, Mung, raw	1 cup	30	3	6	na	4	t	t/0	0	na	15
Squash, spaghetti, boiled or baked, drained, w/o salt	½ cup	21	t	5	1	2	t	t/0	0	14	na
Summer squash, all varieties, sliced, boiled, drained, w/o/ salt	½ cup	18	1	4	1	na	t	t/0	0	1	15
Summer squash, all varieties, sliced, raw	1 cup	23	1	5	2	1.5	t	t/0	0	2	15
Summer squash, crookneck and straightneck, diced, canned	½ cup	14	t	3	1.5	1.5	t	t/0	0	5	15
Summer squash, crookneck and straightneck, mashed, canned, w/o salt	½ cup	16	1	4	2	1	t	t/0	0	6	15
Summer squash, crookneck and straightneck, slices, canned, w/o salt	½ cup	14	t	3	1.5	1	t	t/0	0	5	15
Summer squash, crookneck and straightneck, frozen, w/o salt	½ cup	24	1	5	1	1	t	t/0	0	6	15

Food	Serving	Cal	Prot (g)	Carb (g)	Fiber (g)	Sugars (g)	Total Fat (g)	Sat/Trans Fat (g)	Chol (g)	Sod (mg)	GI
Summer squash, crookneck and straightneck, slices, raw	1 cup	25	1	5	2.5	1	t	t/0	0	3	15
Succotash, boiled, drained, w/o salt	½ cup	110	5	23	4	na	t	t/0	0	16	15
Succotash, frozen, boiled, drained, w/o salt	½ cup	79	4	17	3.5	na	t	t/0	0	38	na
Sweet potato, baked in skin, w/o salt	½ cup	103	2	24	3	7	t	t/0	0	10	50
Sweet potato, baked in skin, w/o salt	1 medium	117	2	28	3	7	t	t/0	0	11	50
Sweet potato, canned, mashed	½ cup	129	3	30	2	6	t	t/0	0	96	50
Sweet potatoes, frozen, cubes, baked, w/o salt	½ cup	88	1	21	2	8	t	t/0	0	7	50
Taro shoots, slices, cooked, w/o salt	½ cup	10	t	2	na	na	t	t/0	0	1	na
Taro shoots, slices, raw	1 cup	9	1	2	na	na	t	t/0	0	1	na
Turnips, cubes, boiled, drained, w/o salt	½ cup	16	t	4	1.5	2	t	0/0	2	na	85

Food	Serving	Cal	Prot (g)	Carb (g)	Fiber (g)	Sugars (g)	Total Fat (g)	Sat/Trans Fat (g)	Chol (g)	Sod (mg)	GI
Turnips, mashed, boiled, drained, w/o salt	½ cup	24	1	6	1.5	2	t	0/0	2	na	85
Turnips, frozen, boiled, drained, w/o salt	½ cup	18	1	3	1.5	2	t	0/0	2	na	85
Turnip greens and turnips, frozen, boiled, drained, w/o salt	½ cup	15	2	2	1.5	1	t	0/0	1.5	na	13
Vegetables, mixed, canned	½ cup	38	2	8	5	2	t	0/0	2	na	na
Vegetables, mixed, frozen, boiled, drained, w/salt	½ cup	54	3	12	4	3	t	0/0	4	121	na
Vegetables, mixed, frozen, boiled, drained, w/o salt	½ cup	54	3	12	4	3	t	0/0	4	na	32
Water chestnuts, Chinese, slices, canned	½ cup	35	t	9	na	na	t	0/0	2	na	6
Watercress, chopped, raw	1 cup	4	1	t	t	t	t	0/0	t	na	14
Watercress, raw	10 sprigs	3	t	t	t	t	t	0/0	t	na	10
Winter squash, all varieties, baked, w/o salt	½ cup	40	1	9	3	3	t	t/0	0	1	na

Food	Serving	Cal	Prot (g)	Carb (g)	Fiber (g)	Sugars (g)	Total Fat (g)	Sat/Trans Fat (g)	Chol (g)	Sod (mg)	GI
Yams, cooked w/salt	½ cup	78	1	18	3	t	t	0/0	0	166	50
Yams, cooked w/o salt	½ cup	78	1	18	3	t	t	0/0	0	5	50
Zucchini, frozen, boiled, drained, w/o salt	½ cup	19	1	4	1	1.5	t	0/0	1	na	2
Zucchini, sliced, boiled, drained, w/o salt	½ cup	14	t	4	1	1.5	t	0/0	1	na	3
Zucchini, mashed, boiled, drained, w/o salt	½ cup	19	1	5	2	2	t	0/0	2	na	4
Zucchini, chopped, raw	1 cup	17	1	4	1	2	t	0/0	1.5	na	4
VEGETABLE JUICES											
Carrot juice, canned	1 cup	94	2	22	2	9	t	t/0	0	68	43
Clam and tomato juice	1 can (5.5 oz)	80	1	18	t	5.5	t	t/0	0	601	na
Mixed vegetable and fruit juice drink	1 serving	110	t	28	t	5	t		0	20	na
Tomato juice, w/o salt	1 cup	41	2	10	2	9	t	t/0	0	24	38
Tomato juice, w/salt	1 cup	41	2	10	1	9	t	t/0	0	877	38

Food	Serving	Cal	Prot (g)	Carb (g)	Fiber (g)	Sugars (g)	Total Fat (g)	Sat/Trans Fat (g)	Chol (g)	Sod (mg)	GI
Vegetable juice cocktail, canned	1 cup	46	1.5	11	2	8	t	t/0	0	653	43
YOGURT											
Fruit-flavored, creamy style, low-fat (1% milkfat)	1 cup	232	9	45	20	45	2	1	39	125	14–33
Fruit-flavored, low-fat (1% milkfat)	1 cup	218	9	41	20	41	2	1	39.50	118	14–33
Fruit-flavored, whole fat	1 cup	252	11	38	13	38	6	2	na	156	36
Frozen yogurt, chocolate, soft serve	½ cup	115	3	18	4	8	4	3	na	71	56–69
Frozen yogurt, vanilla, soft serve	½ cup	114	3	17	1	8	4	2.5	na	63	56–69
Frozen yogurt, hard, low-fat, all flavors	½ cup	140	2.5	26	na	18	3	na	na	na	56–69
Frozen yogurt, nonfat, w/ low-calorie sweetener	½ cup	100	4	18	2	12	1	t	3	75	56–69
Light yogurt (Yoplait)	6 oz	100	5	19	0	14	0	0	t	85	33
Nonfat, no-sugar yogurt, vanilla, lemon, maple, or coffee flavor	1 cup	105	10	18	0	0	t	t	5	144	23

Food	Serving	Cal	Prot (g)	Carb (g)	Fiber (g)	Sugars (g)	Total Fat (g)	Sat/Trans Fat (g)	Chol (g)	Sod (mg)	GI
Nonfat yogurt, strawberry, w/aspartame and fructose (Kraft Breyers Light)	1 cup	125	8	22	0	17	t	t	11	102	23
Plain yogurt, low-fat	1 cup	143	12	16	0	na	4	2	14	159	23
Plain yogurt, skim milk	1 cup	127	13	17	0	17	t	t	5	175	23
Plain, whole milk	1 cup	179	19	11	na	11	7	na	na	na	35
Yogurt fruit smoothies, bottled	1 bottle (10 fl oz)	270	8	52	15	0	3.5	2	50	130	na

REFERENCES

Adler, A.I. Lower prevalence of impaired glucose tolerance and diabetes associated with daily seal oil or salmon consumption among Alaska Natives. *Diabetes Care* 17:1498–1501, 1994.

American Diabetes Association. Standards of Medical Care in Diabetes—2007. *Diabetes Care* 30:S3, 2007.

Coyne, T., et al. Diabetes mellitus and serum carotenoids: findings of a population-based study in Queensland, Australia. *American Journal of Clinical Nutrition* 82:685–693, 2005.

Diabetes Prevention Program Research Group. Reduction in the incidence of type 2 diabetes with lifestyle intervention or metformin. *New England Journal of Medicine* 346:393–403, 2002.

Foster-Powell K., and J.B. Miller. International tables of glycemic index. *American Journal of Clinical Nutrition* 62:871S–890S, 1995.

Garg, A., et al. High-monounsaturated fat diet for diabetic patients. Is it time to change the current dietary recommendations? *Diabetes Care* 17:242–246, 1994.

Gross, L.S., et al. Increased consumption of refined carbohydrates and the epidemic of type 2 diabetes in the United States: an ecologic assessment. *American Journal of Clinical Nutrition* 79:774–779, 2004.

Iso, H., et al. The relationship between green tea and

total caffeine intake and risk for self-reported type 2 diabetes among Japanese adults. *Annals of Internal Medicine* 144:554–562, 2006.

Jiang, R., et al. Nut and peanut butter consumption and risk of type 2 diabetes in women. *Journal of the American Medical Association* 288:2,554–2,560, 2002.

Leitzmann, C. Vegetarian diets: what are the advantages? *Forum of Nutrition* 57:147–156, 2005.

Liu, S., et al. A prospective study of dairy intake and the risk of type 2 diabetes in women. *Diabetes Care* 29:1,579–1,584, 2006.

Lopez-Ridaura, R., et al. Magnesium intake and risk of type 2 diabetes in men and women. *Diabetes Care* 27:134–140, 2004.

Miller, J.C. Importance of glycemic index in diabetes. *American Journal of Clinical Nutrition* 59:747S–752S, 1994.

Schulz, L.O., et al. Effects of traditional and western environments on prevalence of type 2 diabetes in Pima Indians in Mexico and the U.S. *Diabetes Care* 29:1,866–1,871, 2006.

Song, Y., et al. A prospective study of red meat consumption and type 2 diabetes in middle-aged and elderly women: the women's health study. *Diabetes Care* 27:2,108–2,115, 2004.

Wannamethee, S.G., et al. Alcohol drinking patterns and risk of type 2 diabetes mellitus among younger women. *Archives of Internal Medicine* 163:1,329–1,336, 2003.